Unselfish
COURAGE

Kathy Tusen
Schneider

Unselfish
COURAGE

by Kathy Tuson

Pentland Press, Inc.
England • USA •Scotland

PUBLISHED BY PENTLAND PRESS, INC.
5122 Bur Oak Circle, Raleigh, North Carolina 27612
United States of America
919-782-0281
ISBN 1-57197-105-X

Library of Congress Catalog Card Number 97-075986
Copyright © 1996 Kathy Tuson

For

Shelley

&

Special Thanks To

My Parents Owen and Lois Kiely
Who Have Given Me a Lifetime
of
Unconditional Love

Acknowledgments

This Story would not have been possible without the support of family, friends, clergy and Healthcare professionals who shared our battle against cancer. I love you all.

Special thanks to Karen Anderson, Martha Thompson, Suzanne Wilson and Kost Elisevich, M.D., Ph.D. who edited my first drafts and encouraged me to pursue publication.

Prologue

Tuesday, July 20, 1993, is a date I will never forget. What happened on this day changed my life forever.

On Monday, July 19, some girl friends had come over for dinner. We were laughing and enjoying the new hot tub that my husband, Tracey, just had to have. I thought it had been an extravagance, but he wore me down with his persistence and convinced me that it had true therapeutic value.

Tracey came home about 9 P.M. and was subdued because his physician had scheduled a CAT scan. The previous week we had noticed symptoms, slurred speech and a droop in the corner of his lip. They were similar to problems that he had the year before when he had been diagnosed with Bell's palsy. He was worried. I was confident that nothing was wrong. He was forty-three years old and healthy as a horse. He had started taking steroids, and the symptoms had practically disappeared. The CAT scan was just a precaution. I had a sales call in South Bend, Indiana the next day, so I woke at 4 A.M. on Tuesday, July 20, to catch an early bird flight. The meetings lasted all day, and I waited until 10 P.M. that evening to call Tracey. The phone rang twice, and a hushed voice answered. I knew immediately that something was terribly wrong. He began to cry. Tracey had cried only one other time during our relationship.

The doctor had called early that morning. We needed to make an appointment with a neurosurgeon. He had a brain tumor.

The story that follows will make you cry. It will make you laugh. But most of all, I hope that by sharing the details of our experience, you will treasure the love you receive because love is life . . . and if you miss love, you miss life.

Chapter One

Not Love at First Sight

When Tracey and I met, we seemed to have very little in common. He was gregarious; I was reserved. He golfed and snow skied; I played tennis, softball, and racquetball. He looked young; I looked younger. What we did share was a sense of humor, a competitive spirit, a group of mutual friends, and a desire to enjoy life.

I was president of a snow ski club. This might lead you to ask the question, "If she played tennis, softball, and racquetball, why is she president of a ski club?" There is a perfectly logical explanation. First, I joined the club to play in a racquetball league, and second, they elected me by a unanimous vote. You see, I was very popular—which means that no one else wanted the job.

We met on the phone. Tracey called me to ask a question about the next monthly meeting. He introduced himself as a ski racer. He acted as if I should know him because he was some kind of jock. I was a little put off, but he had my attention. Who was this guy who thought that "moi," as Miss Piggy would say, the president (I had my ego), should know who he was? I was definitely curious. At the next meeting, I was standing by the entrance and recognized his voice, as I have this uncanny memory for voices. I walked up to him and blurted out, "You must be Tracey Tuson." He looked a little befuddled and didn't know quite what to say. I chatted with him for thirty seconds and then ran off. After all, I was the president. I had things to do and people to meet. It definitely was not love at first sight. In fact, my first impression was, "He's nothing special." A year later he told me that initially he thought that I was a tall, dumb blonde. I was flabbergasted. Tall and blond, okay, but I had never in my life been described as dumb. I was a Phi Beta Kappa and had graduated summa cum laude. For God's sake, I had a master's degree. Why would he ever be interested in me if I were dumb? He simply laughed and said, "Dumb can be fun!" Luckily, I couldn't read his mind when we met or I wouldn't have given him the time of day.

A month after our first encounter, our paths happened to cross. We were both snow skiing at Boyne Mountain in northern Michigan. Tracey would vehemently disagree, but I did know how to ski. It's just that some people would call it an advanced snow plow. Our club was sponsoring Carnival Weekend. As president, I was responsible for coordinating a ski race, a dance, and other events. It was an easy way to raise money and have fun at the same time. We entered an inner-tube race together in which I was slammed into a snow fence because Tracey, who abandoned ship just as we crossed the finish line, wanted to win. I like to win but didn't relish being killed in the process. Strike one for Tracey. Saturday night there was a dance. Even though dancing was one of my favorite things to do, I had other priorities. I was very busy checking on everything, collecting money, and solving problems. Tracey was busy selling beer. I think he served more beer than he drank, but I'm not sure. All evening he pestered me for a dance. It couldn't be just any dance. It had to be a slow dance. In order to placate him, I promised, "I'll dance with you later. I'm just too busy right now." It seemed like every time I stopped for a moment, Tracey was tapping me on the shoulder and wanted to know, "How about now?" I had never been pursued so ardently. It was very clear to me that he was infatuated, but since we barely knew one another, I was confused by his behavior. I thought to myself, "He doesn't know anything about me. Why is he acting like this?" I didn't know what to make of him. I decided that he was different, and definitely persistent. About midnight, things slowed down and for the first time that evening, I danced with a good friend. As soon as the music stopped, I heard a voice behind me say, "I thought you said that you were too busy." Tracey finally had me cornered. We had barely started to dance when the music

changed. Everybody else began to hop to the new tempo.
Everybody but Tracey. He held onto me and continued to slow
dance. I glanced around at the other people and whispered,
"Trace, you can slow dance to anything, can't you?" He just
grinned and nodded.

On Sunday, my friends who had given me a ride to Boyne
Mountain for the weekend wanted to leave early. I had to stay
until late afternoon because of my responsibilities. While I was
talking to some friends about my problem, I saw Tracey. I
hesitated for a moment. I generally didn't ask strangers for help,
but I was in a bind. He seemed harmless. Maybe he wouldn't
mind. Tracey jumped at the chance. Here I had been avoiding
him all weekend, and suddenly he would have my undivided
attention for five hours. There was a God after all! Little did he
know that I planned to sleep the whole way home. I was
exhausted and could hardly keep my eyes open. For the first half
hour, Tracey sneezed and coughed so much that I was afraid that
we were going to end up in a ditch. He had a terrible cold, so I
offered to drive. He politely declined my offer because he didn't
trust anyone else driving. They might fall asleep, which was
exactly my plan. Unfortunately for me, that was not Tracey's
plan. He talked nonstop for the entire five hour drive. I have a
great sense of humor, but I was not easily amused by most men.
Tracey, on the other hand, told stories and jokes that made me
laugh. Before I knew it, we were at my house and I hadn't had
my nap. I remember thanking him for the ride and saying good-
bye. As I entered my living room, I was shaking my head and
mumbling to myself, "That boy can talk!"

For the next six months, we saw each other at the monthly
ski club meetings. I could tell that Tracey was still very interested
in me, but I kept him at arm's length. I was dating two other men
and taking two graduate classes. There just wasn't any time for
anyone else in my life. He discovered that I loved ice cream and
convinced me to go with him on our first date to Baskin-Robbins.
We had a good time just talking with each other, and Tracey
suggested meeting for lunch the following day. It was his day off,
so we met at a restaurant close to my job. After eating lunch, we
went back to my house which was close by. We sat on the couch,
and he leaned over to kiss me. It was then that every man's
dream came true. My clothes started to fall off. I generally didn't
wear this particular blouse without a jacket or a sweater. You
only had to touch it and all the buttons down the back popped
open. As Tracey brought his arm around me, every button came

undone, one after another, like a stack of dominoes tumbling down. Our first kiss came to an abrupt halt. Tracey was embarrassed and at a loss for words. Here he had been trying to impress me with how he could be a gentleman, and fate was against him. He thought that I would never see him again. I was laughing to myself but did not say anything. For such a competitive jock and long winded talker, his reaction revealed a rather shy, romantic side which surprised and amused me. Since I needed to return to work, Tracey excused himself and said he'd call me later. I guess I have an evil streak in me because I didn't tell him about that blouse until we were married.

Over the next two years, we became inseparable. Tracey decided that I needed to learn how to ski and golf. I insisted that he join my tennis club. We both loved sports and enjoyed doing them together. After four months, Tracey told me that he loved me. But it was a full year before I could say, "I love you," to him. I had only said those three simple words to one other person in my life, other than my family, and that had ended in divorce. It was not something that I had allowed myself to say, let alone feel. I wasn't sure that I could ever love or trust anyone again. But Tracey was breaking down my barriers. He was fun and made me laugh. However, what affected me the most was that he wanted to know everything about me. It was not in my nature to share personal feelings easily, but he questioned me until he was able to open doors that I thought were forever locked. From the very start of our relationship, Tracey was not shy about expressing his affection for me both verbally and nonverbally. Frequently at parties, I could feel his eyes following me as I moved around the room. It was very scary to be loved because of the painful memories from my previous marriage. Gradually, however, I realized that I had fallen deeply in love.

We took vacations together, and I grew to know his daughter, Shelley. She was a wonderful little girl. She was so much like him and loved him so much. I started to want to belong to a family. I wanted my own family. What happens in so many relationships happened to us. We found ourselves in two different emotional places. I wanted more. I wanted to get married.

Tracey was also divorced and was afraid of commitment. He didn't want to lose me, but he kept changing his mind about getting married. We started to argue because I felt that Tracey wasn't being honest with me. For the next six months, we saw each other on again, off again. Finally, I had enough. If Tracey couldn't make a decision, I would. I told him to leave me alone.

If he saw me, he was to ignore me because I planned to ignore him. I was devastated. I felt as if he had lied to me. My heart ached, and I had lost all trust once again. It was too painful to love because it did not last—no matter how perfect the match seemed.

For three months, we did not see or talk with one another. I was trying to move on with my life. In December 1984, some friends surreptitiously arranged for us to be at the same Christmas party. They later told us that they knew that we belonged with one another. We just needed a push in the right direction. Tracey followed me around all evening like a little puppy dog. My girl friend noticed Tracey's persistent behavior and asked me, "What's wrong with him? Why won't he leave you alone?" I was irritated and tried to ignore him, but it was useless. I considered leaving, but my stubborn streak said, "Don't let him ruin your good time." I was uncomfortable and started drinking Long Island iced tea that was being served from a punch bowl. As I was leaving at the end of the evening, Tracey asked if he could walk me to my car. Maybe it was the liquor, but I think that I was just curious. What did he want? As we approached my car, he took my hand and began to cry. He apologized, "Kathy, I'm so sorry. I've made a terrible mistake. I need you in my life. Will you marry me?" I was in shock. For a moment, neither one of us said a word. Tracey was waiting for my answer. I looked him in the eye and said, "I know that I still love you, but I hate you for what you've done to me. I don't know if I can ever trust you again." Tracey had knocked at my door, but I couldn't remove the chain. The words "I love you," seemed to come too easily for Tracey. I agreed to meet him the next day and talk. For the next four months, we worked on rebuilding our relationship. One day, Tracey was holding me and said, "Something has changed. I feel like I've lost you." I didn't reply but I thought to myself, "Yes, you're right. But I hope that you search long enough to find me." He did, and in March 1985, during the Carnival Ski Weekend at Boyne Mountain, we became engaged.

We were married October 6, 1985. A couple of years later, Tracey confessed that he had been worried the day we were married. He was afraid that when the wedding was over, I would change and wouldn't be fun anymore. I laughed at him and shook my head. What we didn't realize was that we would both change, for over the next ten years, our friendship and love would grow beyond anything that we ever anticipated.

It had always been a mutual dream to live on the water. We bought a house on a lake and learned how to water-ski. We were able to maintain old friendships that we had developed through snow skiing and golf, but we made many new acquaintances through water skiing. We were very happy. We were like two peas in a pod. Shelley even commented one day that, "You guys are so much alike it's scary."

This is not to say that our lives were perfect. We worked very hard at our relationship. Although they were infrequent, we did have a few major confrontations. However, we talked about everything, and our first priority was always our marriage and family. We knew that no matter what happened, nothing could come between us as long as we had each other's best interests at heart.

Beginning in 1992, the company that Tracey worked for tried to convince long term employees to retire or take a buyout. Pressure was mounting, but he did not want to leave. Tracey had been with Sears for almost twenty years, and he was consistently one of the top salespeople. On Tuesday, July 20, 1993, instead of deciding on a career change, Tracey received the results of his CAT scan and took a medical leave of absence.

Chapter Two
Finding Help

"I HAVE A BRAIN TUMOR." Even though he whispered softly, his words screamed in my ears. Denial. It can't be true. It's a mistake. What do I do? My mind raced. I have to get home right away. Tracey was alone, isolated, and afraid. He was paralyzed with fear and had not talked to anyone. He needed me and I had left town. I had deserted him when he needed me the most. We talked for five minutes. Although he told me he was okay, I knew that I could not wait until the next day to fly back. In five hours, I would be home. In the meantime, Tracey needed to talk with someone. I called a friend, John, who is a doctor. I blurted out the horrible news to his wife, Wendy. Yes, John would go to our house and stay with Tracey.

The drive home was a blur. How could this be happening? It wasn't fair! I had waited too long to love and be loved. I was not going to lose my husband, my lover, my best friend. We were supposed to grow old together. We had plans! When I unlocked the door at 3 A.M., the house was still. I ran upstairs. Tracey was sleeping, or perhaps he was only resting his eyes. I climbed into bed and wrapped my arms around him and began to weep softly. We would face this nightmare tomorrow. Tonight, my need to hold him was as great as his to be held.

Tracey had talked to our friend, John, and felt he had received good advice—get a couple of opinions. John would help if we needed him. Tracey's internist had given him a referral. However, when we called the neurosurgeon's office on Wednesday morning, the receptionist told us that we would have to wait two weeks for an appointment. Fortunately, I was angry and swung into action. Tracey once described me as being relentless. On this day, this characteristic would be an asset, not a liability. I telephoned Tracey's internist and persuaded him to intervene. He personally called the same neurosurgeon and soon we had an appointment for Friday.

RULE #1—ASK YOUR FRIENDS AND FAMILY FOR HELP! My cousin, Jake, worked for Henry Ford Health Systems, and put me touch with Ardis Gregory, who was part of a customer service support hotline for the hospital. She collected background information, cut through all the administrative red tape, and within three hours, we had an appointment with another neurosurgeon for the next afternoon. I talked with friends who gave me the names of other doctors. For good measure, I called a third specialist and left a message. Now, we had to wait. Waiting was going to become a major part of our life for the next twenty-eight months.

Fear is a strange phenomenon. It can paralyze you. Tracey was in shock and was unable to think clearly. From this point in our life, I became Tracey's advocate in every sense of the word. I was like a lioness who would protect her cub at any cost. I would be his ears when he could not listen, his voice when he could not speak, and his eyes when he could not bear to see. We would share our strength and love with each other in ways that I never knew were possible.

On Thursday, July 22, 1993, at 3 P.M., we had our first consultation at Henry Ford Hospital. With x-ray film in hand, we were escorted to an examining room and were told that Dr. Elisevich would be with us shortly. I think that we were still in a state of denial, because we were both nonchalantly leafing through magazines. Apparently, we appeared to be too calm because when the neurosurgeon looked in, he thought he was in the wrong room. Couldn't he hear our hearts pounding in our chests? Couldn't he see the fear in our eyes? We heard the nurse say, "No, that's the right room." Kost Elisevich not only entered the room, but he also entered our lives.

He was dressed in green scrubs and looked very young— almost too young. My first impression was, "Not another Doogie Howser, M.D.!" How many years did it take to become a neurosurgeon? How much experience could he possibly have? Is he the best? Could we trust him? Would he be insulted if I asked him for his resume? All these thoughts crossed our minds as he introduced himself. "Hello! I'm Kost Elisevich." We shook hands. He sat toe-to-toe with Tracey and carelessly tossed the x-ray on the table. He locked eyes with Tracey and said, "I've looked at your scans, but what I really want to know about is you." Within thirty seconds, we felt like we had a friend, even though he still looked awfully young. For the next forty-five minutes, Kost— yes, we called him by his first name; isn't that what friends do?— listened, asked questions, and calmed our fears. It could be an abscess. It could be a tumor. The only way to find out was surgery. What would be involved? What were the risks?

Physicians are very clever people. They know that if they scare you too much, you will run. So they all describe "the procedure" the same way. We create a small window (not a "bay window" or a "door wall"), remove the abnormal tissue (not "large tumor mass"), and determine what it is. He warned us that as with any surgery, problems arise. However, he felt that there was only a one or two percent chance that Tracey would lose any functionality. Every physician we saw said, "create a small window" and "the risk is minimal." There must be certain phrases that they teach doctors in medical school. Maybe we were afraid, but we never asked, "What do you mean, create a small window?" We just accepted what they said. Since they all said the same thing, it would be okay. At least they were consistent.

At times of extreme stress, humor takes over my thought processes. My imagination runs wild. All I could picture was the surgeon opening a little trap door on the side of Tracey's head, peeking in, and saying "S'all right?" A little voice would echo back "S'all right." The trap door would snap shut, and we would go home healthy and happy. Some people will think that my humor is sick, but I was able to laugh at myself instead of becoming hysterical. I did discover, however, that once you become a patient, the real confusion starts. You must carry a dictionary at all times, unless of course, you can afford a full-time medical terminology interpreter.

We thought that we understood what would be involved. It's amazing how naive intelligent people can be. We had no idea what was in store for us. We told Kost that we were getting a second opinion the following day. He immediately agreed, and said that there were many excellent neurosurgeons. However, he cautioned us that we should not delay making a decision. He introduced us to the nurse, Alona Moon, who could help us schedule the surgery, and wished us luck. During our appointment, it seemed as if Kost would have spent the entire afternoon with us if we needed him. It seemed as if we were the center of his universe. However, as we watched him rush down the hallway, it was evident that he was very busy.

Our next appointment was Friday, July 23, at 11 A.M. First impressions are significant and become critical when important decisions need to be made. Before we even met the next neurosurgeon, we were offended. We were required to sign a statement acknowledging that we understood that we were liable for any and all fees no matter what insurance we had. We were there for a $150 opinion, not a major life commitment. We felt that we were dollar signs instead of people. Things did not improve. The neurosurgeon was delayed, and Tracey was asked to disrobe for no reason. When he finally arrived, the physician apologized but continually looked at his watch. His recommendation was basically the same, and he was with us for forty-five minutes. However, it seemed as if he couldn't wait to get to the next patient. When we mentioned that we wanted another opinion, he seemed offended and warned us about selecting a teaching hospital, because Tracey would probably be treated by residents. We knew that this physician had a good reputation and was attempting to be helpful, but we were totally turned off by his bedside manner.

We had to make a choice. Both physicians seemed competent and stressed the need to operate as soon as possible. We could not procrastinate. It felt like we were waiting for a SWAT team to diffuse a ticking time bomb which could explode at any moment. We liked and felt comfortable with Kost Elisevich. But he looked so young. Was he a resident? We telephoned Alona Moon who scheduled surgery for Kost. Unknowingly, she helped us make our decision. Realizing that we needed to be confident before making this life decision, she confirmed that Kost was not a resident, and simply said, "He is world class." Nurses don't exaggerate their opinions about doctors. Our minds were made up. After spending only forty-five minutes with a total stranger, Tracey entrusted his life into a pair of hands that created a new window in our lives.

Chapter Three

Surgery

Surgery was scheduled for Thursday, July 29, 1993. Six days to wait. It seemed like an eternity. There were two days of prerequisite tests, a physical exam, bloodwork, and x-rays, which the neurosurgeon required. He wanted to make sure that there were no surprises during or after surgery. What we didn't realize was that they wanted to make sure that there were no tumors elsewhere in Tracey's body. Since many people were involved in performing these tests, there was an extraordinary amount of scheduling that needed to occur. This is when I realized how lucky we were that the people on whom we were depending were dedicated and compassionate.

We chose Kost as our neurosurgeon at noon on Friday, July 23. All of the tests needed to be completed by Monday, July 26, in order for the surgery to take place the following Thursday. Alona Moon needed to schedule everything, and she was leaving for her vacation at the end of the day. She only had four hours before she left. I don't know how she arranged everything in such a short period of time, because it took a number of phone calls, asking favors, and completing volumes of paperwork. But by the end of the day Friday, we knew that surgery would happen the next week. We experienced this level of help many times over the next two years. I will be forever grateful to Alona and the many other people who helped us, not simply because it was their job, but because we needed them.

Surgery is frightening to most people. Tracey wanted to get it over with as soon as possible. It couldn't happen soon enough for him. We used the next week to prepare ourselves and our families. As you can imagine, Tracey was in a state of shock, and needed to conserve his energy to face an unknown enemy. If you ever watched the movie, "Brian's Song," you will remember the scene where the doctor asks Brian Piccolo, a football player diagnosed with cancer, to sign a surgery release. He refuses. Gayle Sayers, a teammate and friend, intervenes and tells the doctor that "Brian needs to prepare himself." He explains that some athletes need space and time to build their inner strength before every big game. Tracey was building his inner strength. He could not waste any emotion on anyone. As his advocate, I took the responsibility for breaking the news to everyone. The most difficult part was not being able to tell people what they wanted to hear—that there is nothing to worry about, that Tracey will be okay, that he will not die! I could only tell them what I knew, which was that the doctor would create a small window, and the risk is minimal. Everyone wanted to help, but there was nothing anyone could do, except be our friend and pray. We felt helpless.

Tracey and I were both afraid of this surgery. But he feared being left alone, being deserted. I didn't understand this fear, but tried to reassure him that I would never leave him. Eight years ago, I had made a sacred vow to love him in sickness and in health. Nothing had changed. No matter what happened, I would always love him. Didn't he know that he was part of my heart and soul? It wasn't until much later that I realized I too feared being left alone—deserted—by his death.

While we waited for the day of the operation to arrive, I stayed home with Tracey, and we spent time together. Since it was summer, we were able to water-ski, which was a wonderful distraction. Sports had always been the way that we relaxed. For short periods of time, we were able to forget everything that was bothering us. We definitely needed to maintain a positive attitude in order to keep our sanity. Thursday seemed so far away, but those few days passed too quickly. There was not enough time to do the things that we had dreamed of doing. So instead, we made sure that we told each other everything that needed to be said. No words were left unspoken. We loved one another.

The night before his surgery, Shelley, Tracey's daughter, spent the night. A nineteen year old college student, she lived thirty minutes away with her mother. She wanted to be with her dad. We woke up at 4 A.M. on Thursday morning, because we needed to be at the hospital by 6 A.M. Tracey was quietly getting ready. Twice I tried to wake Shelley, and then realized that there was a problem. She was diabetic and was having an insulin reaction. My heart started to pound. What do I do? She was incoherent, but able to walk. We went to the kitchen, where I made sure she drank a Coke and ate a donut. I called her mom, Connie, in a panic. She talked calmly with me, even though I know her heart was pounding too. I described Shelley's symptoms. Luckily, it only took a few moments for Shelley to come around. She would probably be very tired and fall asleep, but she would be okay. Tracey was oblivious to what was happening. Thank God he was in his own little world. We climbed into the car for the first of many trips to Henry Ford Hospital.

When we arrived, I felt like we were on an assembly line. Sign here. Go there. Wait. At 6:15 A.M., with tears in my eyes, I kissed Tracey Tuson good-bye. I was afraid that I would never see him again. Since he would be in intensive care, they wanted me to wait and take his personal belongings. About twenty minutes later, they gave me his clothes and a small, brown paper bag that was sealed. I looked a little confused and the nurse said, "We saved his hair that needed to be shaved off for surgery." Now I was really concerned that I would never see him again. This small bag of hair might be all that I had left of him after surgery. My heart sank.

We wandered off to the waiting room and registered with the attendant. The surgery would be over by noon. Two or three times during the operation, a nurse would talk to me by phone and let me know the status of the surgery. I brought a book, but I could not read. I was tired, but I could not sleep. I was restless, but I could not leave. So I sat. Tracey's parents joined us in the waiting room. We were all nervous. I noticed that there were other families just sitting too. We all had the same stoic look on our faces. We started to talk to one another, to console one another, and to congratulate one another when a loved one's surgery was over. We had nothing in common, yet we had everything in common. We were afraid that we would lose someone we loved.

At 9:30 A.M. I jumped when I was paged to take a call. I ran to the phone, even though I dreaded bad news. Then I realized that if anything terrible had happened, they would not call me on the phone and say, "I'm sorry Mrs. Tuson. Your husband just died." Instead, a comforting voice said, "Everything is going well. We have just completed 'creating the window,' and the surgical procedure is just about to begin. It will be at least another hour before we have more news. Why don't you get some breakfast?" There was that damn window again! I thought to myself, "Oh yeah! Let me run right down and order some bacon, hash browns, and eggs—over easy." But the nurse was right. We needed a break. So we went to the cafeteria. I'm not sure what everyone else ate, but the only thing I thought I could hold down was some yogurt.

When the next phone call came, I was not as apprehensive. The surgery was over, and Tracey had done well. Kost would be out in thirty minutes to talk with us. What a relief! Tracey was alive.

I anxiously watched surgeons come and go. Some physicians casually talked to families in the middle of the waiting room. Didn't these doctors know that families needed privacy? Small conference rooms were available but not used. We were luckier than some of the families that I watched. I saw Kost enter the room and hurried toward him. Before he could say anything, I grasped his hand and thanked him. He smiled and directed us to one of the small conference rooms. He sat toe-to-toe with me, because I was now the patient. His eyes bored into me as if he were looking for something. He described the surgery and drew pictures. He was not a great artist, but he got the point across, and that was all that mattered. The surgery was a success, and the patient lived. They were still not sure whether the growth was an abscess, and probably would not know for a few days. Just in case, he was prescribing antibiotics which would be administered intravenously.

They had also taken a look at some tissue samples. There did not appear to be any traces of melanoma. (Medical Terminology 101 had begun. Where was my medical dictionary when I needed it?) From somewhere in my memory, I recalled that melanoma meant cancer. I felt like I was in a state of suspended animation. I heard my father-in-law gasp, and I felt tears flow from my eyes. Kost touched my hand to comfort me. I reacted by pulling back. I was not used to being touched by strangers. He had entered my comfort zone unexpectedly, and it startled me. I quickly came back to reality and realized that Tracey still had a chance. He might escape the grip of cancer. Now, we had to wait for the test results. If the tissue cultures grew, the growth was an infection. Otherwise, the pathology report would analyze and identify the tissue. Would it be cancer? The SWAT team was not finished. The bomb was still ticking. My attention focused on Kost. It was my turn to look into his eyes. I thanked him not only for his skill as a surgeon, but for his compassion as a human being. He had given us a sense of security and the gifts of hope and trust. He had calmed Tracey's spirit. We would soon find out that he had given us much more—he had given us his unselfish courage.

Chapter Four

Recovery

For the next five hours, we waited for Tracey to be moved to intensive care. We were becoming impatient and concerned. Was something wrong? Fortunately, there was good communication with the staff in recovery. There was a delay because there were not any available beds in ICU. Finally, Tracey was transported and we were able to see him. I was expecting the worst, but he actually looked good. His cheeks were pink, and his head was wrapped in a bandage. The white gauze almost looked like a mushroom cap. The nurse called Tracey's name a few times, and his eyes opened. I was holding his hand and leaned over and lightly kissed him on the lips. His eyes filled with tears and he whispered, "I love you." I felt like they were the sweetest words that I had ever heard. He wanted to know the outcome of his surgery, and I told him that they had been able to remove all visible signs of the growth. I moved away so that Shelley and Tracey's parents could talk with him. We were there about five minutes and he closed his eyes. It had been a long day. I told everyone to go home and come back the next day. There were signs to limit visits to two people for short periods of time. But the nursing staff allowed me to stay so that I could just hold his hand. I know I needed his touch as much as he needed mine. I stayed for another four hours. During this time, I was amazed by how busy the nurses were. They had forms to fill out, medications to dispense, vital signs to check, and machines to monitor. Every so often, they woke Tracey and asked him questions. Tracey knew that he was being tested. He wanted to prove that he was healthy, to pass their tests so that he'd be discharged as soon as possible. They were fairly straightforward questions like, "What's your name? Where are you? Why are you here? What day is it?" Tracey passed with flying colors, except when they finally stumped him by asking, "Who is the president?" He closed his eyes, and I could tell that he was thinking very hard. A nurse continued taking Tracey's blood pressure. Suddenly, he gestured with his index finger for the nurse to come close. He whispered something in her ear, and she burst out laughing. I asked what he had said, and she replied, "Hillary." I knew then that Tracey was okay. He still had his sense of humor. I could go home for the night.

I arrived the next morning at 10:30 A.M. Visiting hours did not begin until 11 A.M. While I was waiting, I noticed a minister walking into the ICU. I didn't think much about it until I was visiting Tracey, and noticed a business card from Metropolitan United Methodist Church. Our friends, Diane and Don, had asked one of their clergy, Reverend Bill Wood, to comfort Tracey. This was the first of many visits that we would receive from the ministers of this church. Even though we were not members of the church, they adopted us as part of their Christian family, prayed for us, and became our friends.

I had only seen Tracey for a couple of minutes when he announced he had a funny story to tell. During the night, he had noticed that a concerned doctor had slept in a chair next to a patient. The doctor was so exhausted, that he didn't wake when the nurses put a catheter tube up his pant leg and attached a sign which said "Out of Order." I thanked God that even though this was a place filled with pain and suffering, they still had a sense of humor. It meant that they hadn't cut themselves off emotionally from the patients.

The rest of the day was fairly uneventful except for the parade of physicians who had a sudden interest in Tracey. The "infectious control patrol" had descended. If the abnormal tissue which they had removed and placed in cultures grew, they would need to determine how to fight the infection. They were like Sherlock Holmes in white lab coats. You could see the excitement in their eyes as they asked what seemed like totally ridiculous questions, such as, "Do you have a cat?" After all, it was hard to find a good infectious disease to treat. They departed as they had entered—with thoughtful, questioning eyes.

The nursing staff did an excellent job of limiting visitors. Patients are in the ICU because they need to rest. Sometimes families just get in the way. Most of the day, I sat and visited with the families I had met the day before. It was the first time in my life that I experienced the bond that develops among people who are dealing with the possible death of a loved one. These strangers became my friends. When I cried, they comforted me. When they cried, I wrapped my arms around them. We protected each other. We all needed the touch of another human being.

By late afternoon, Tracey was holding court and entertaining the nurses with his jokes. It was time for him to go to the next level of care, called Step Down. He still needed to be monitored, but didn't need the constant attention of a nurse. However, that's not to say that he didn't want constant attention. He did not want me out of his sight. Tracey was in a semi-private room, so there wasn't much space. I was perched on a radiator next to the bed when Kost walked in at 7 P.M. I was surprised to see him so late in the day, especially on a Friday. He had deep circles under his eyes and looked exhausted. We chatted for a few minutes and then he remarked, "I have to leave for awhile." I looked at him quizzically, and Tracey asked, "Is there something wrong?" He explained that his father had undergone cancer surgery the previous day. Kost told us that he would be gone for two weeks, but other neurosurgeons on staff would take care of Tracey until he was discharged. I was speechless. I was hardly able to say good-bye. His dedication and commitment to his patients were so strong that Kost had not been willing to disappoint us by asking someone else to perform the operation, so that he could be with his father. He was able to set aside his personal needs and focus on a patient who needed him. I was amazed by, and grateful for, his unselfish courage. Weeks later we thanked him, but he looked confused. He remarked, "I couldn't have done anything for my father." In his mind, he hadn't done anything special. Over time, I discovered many exceptional people who helped us with their unselfish courage. What was even more amazing was that no one thought that he or she had done anything special.

At 8 P.M. that day, the head nurse on the floor started clearing out all visitors. She reminded me of a marine drill sergeant. No one dared disobey her orders. It was time for her patients to sleep. Anyone not in bed and hooked to a monitor had to leave.

During the drive home, I cried. Not only was I physically exhausted, but I was mentally drained. I couldn't think anymore. By evening, I was a robot going through the motions. Our message recorder was full. There were always more calls than I had time to answer. All of our friends wanted us to know that they were concerned. I telephoned a few people, and at 11 P.M. crawled into bed. I had just drifted off to sleep when the phone rang. Who could be calling this late? Was it the hospital? An unfamiliar voice said, "Mrs. Tuson, this is Dr. Goodfellow." My heart stopped. "You called me few days ago about your husband. I was out of town and have been trying to reach you. I understand from your message that your husband has a brain tumor. Have you been able to get help?"

I tried to wipe the tears from my cheeks. Dr. Goodfellow, a neurosurgeon from a different hospital, was the third specialist I had called. We had never talked. I thought he had been another doctor who was just too busy to return my phone call. We talked for about twenty minutes. He listened and offered some useful information. As we said good-bye, he gave me his home phone number, "If you need any help or have questions, please call me."

When I woke up on Sunday morning, I was refreshed. A good night's sleep was what I had needed. As I was getting ready to go to the hospital, I had a sudden compulsion to make the bed. Unless we were expecting company, making the bed had never been important to me. When we were first married, I had spent hours convincing Tracey that it was not crucial. Now it had become a priority. What was wrong with me? It bothered me until I realized that the bedroom was the first and last thing I saw every day. I had to keep things tidy because my life was a mess. Making my bed was a small step in helping me gain some control.

When I arrived at the hospital, Tracey was stable. By late morning, he was moved to a private room on the neurological ward. We would have to pay for this luxury, but we decided that we needed more space as well as some peace and quiet. Every day, Tracey was examined by a different physician. They introduced themselves, but we couldn't remember their names. They all looked the same in their white lab coats and green scrubs. During rounds, a decision was made to remove the head bandage. Kost had described the incision, but I felt uneasy as it was slowly unwrapped. Tracey was watching my reaction. I knew I couldn't look away or be upset. I tried to disassociate myself from the fact that I was looking at my husband's head. It worked. Even though he had eighty staples in his head, I made a wisecrack. The incision looked like a big question mark. So I said, "Did they put that punctuation mark on your head because they had a question or what?" As usual, I laughed at my own joke and then proceeded to count the staples. Tracey decided he wanted to look. He stared at himself in a mirror and said, "Maybe I should get a tattoo on my head that says—Bad To The Bone." We agreed that he could get a lot of mileage with this new hairdo. This time we both laughed.

By late Sunday afternoon, there was still no news. I was getting nervous. Tracey was slowly becoming depressed. Hopefully, we would hear something tomorrow. I was beginning to fear the answers that we would receive.

Chapter Five

Diagnosis & Discharge

Remember RULE #1—ASK YOUR FRIENDS FOR HELP! RULE #2 is—RULES ARE MADE TO BE BROKEN! Visiting hours do not begin until 11 A.M., but my intuition told me that Tracey needed me. As I entered the hospital at 9 A.M. on Monday, I told the security guard that the doctor wanted to talk with me. I repeated this half-truth a number of times as I walked to Tracey's room. I knew the doctor wanted to see me, I just didn't know when. Acting confident was all I needed to do. As soon as I saw Tracey, I could see that he was depressed. He looked terrible. His right eye was swollen shut, his face hadn't seen a razor since Thursday, half of his head had been shaved, and the rest of his hair was a greasy mess. There was only one thing to do. He had to take a bath. This was pretty tricky because he had an IV, and the scalp incision could not get wet. Tracey was a modest person, so I thought it would be best if I helped him rather than one of the nursing aides. He needed to maintain his dignity. I changed into my bathing suit so I could climb in the tub with him. The aide saw me prancing around the room in my bathing suit and asked me what I was doing. I told her that I was trying to lift Tracey's spirits, and the rest of the bathing beauties would be in shortly. Tracey chimed in and said that he preferred hot and cold running blondes. I told her that Tracey and I would like to be alone and asked that she close the door on her way out.

She chuckled and left the room. Tracey humored me by agreeing to take a bath. I brought shorts and a T-shirt so that he wouldn't be sitting in a hospital gown all day. My attitude was—if you think you look bad, you feel bad. Once we were done, he felt and looked much better. He took a nap, and we waited for news.

After lunch, a doctor came in and said that they had ruled out an infection because the tissue cultures had not grown. Now we had to wait for the pathology report. I guess this could be considered good news because they were that much closer to figuring out what had caused the growth. But to us, it was not good news. In my mind, an infection was much easier to treat and cure than cancer. Cancer meant death. We wouldn't get another report until Tuesday. Tracey and I did not discuss the ramifications of this news. We were numb with disappointment.

A few friends and family members came, but Tracey was very tired, so they couldn't stay long. It was practically impossible to lift his spirits. He seemed to sink deeper and deeper into himself. The only thing I could do to help was hold his hand. Monday evening I tearfully called John, a friend, who like Tracey, was very athletic but had been fighting to recover from various back and shoulder surgeries. Tracey respected his drive and determination. I thought that a visit from him might help.

By the time I arrived on Tuesday, John had already stopped by and convinced Tracey to walk down the hospital corridor. Tracey had been exhausted after going about one hundred feet, but he was proud of his accomplishment. He even suggested going for another stroll. His energy level was definitely improving.

We watched TV, and late Tuesday afternoon a resident came to give us an update. He was sent on a simple mission: to tell us that the pathology report wouldn't be available until Wednesday. It was at this point that I learned the most important rule of all. RULE #3—NEVER—AND I MEAN NEVER—TALK TO A RESIDENT/INTERN! You have to be very careful about this, because they try to camouflage the fact that they are residents/interns. They introduce themselves as Dr. So-and-So and yet avoid telling you what their position is. Earlier in the day, Dr. So-and-So had checked on Tracey, and he had a confident demeanor. However, when he walked in the room later that day, he looked like a trapped rabbit. The fear in his eyes was very apparent. He slid into the room with his back against the wall. His eyes darted to the doorway. He did not want to be talking with us. No matter what he said, his body language screamed, "Tracey's going to die! Tracey's going to die!" When he felt that he had completed his mission, he could tell that I was not pleased. I'm sure he did not understand why I was perturbed. He justified his hasty departure by saying that the only reason he came to talk with us was due to his earlier promise to return. Luckily, he left because I was ready to rip his heart out. I had a short discussion with a staff member regarding Dr. So-and-So. Fortunately for him and for us, he was never to be seen again during our stay.

On Wednesday, I arrived early again. I was afraid the doctors would tell Tracey bad news without me. I dodged and weaved my way through the various roadblocks without being detected. As long as I was pleasant and quiet, I figured that they would leave me alone. I was right. Around 11 A.M., a doctor whom I remembered from the first day came into the room. He had someone else in tow, who I'm fairly sure was in training, because he was somber and nodded his head at the appropriate moments. The doctor went to Tracey's side and took his hand. I knew at that moment that this was not good. He remarked that they needed to get rid of the IV and asked Tracey if he was ready to go home. Tracey's face lit up for the first time in over a week. Of course he was ready. Then, he talked about the pathology report. He began by saying that the report indicated the growth was the most common type of tumor. Tracey asked, "What kind?" The physician gave the name, anaplastic astrocytoma. It rolled off his tongue like he was saying pizza pie. All I could remember was ana something or another. He then proceeded to inform us that other physicians, an oncologist and a radiation oncologist, had to see us before Tracey could be discharged. Additional treatment was necessary in order to prevent the tumor from recurring. The good news was that this particular type of tumor would not spread anywhere else in the body. It could only grow in the brain. Tracey would be able to leave on Thursday morning. He asked us if we had any questions, but Tracey was in a trance. I felt like Mike Tyson had just punched me in the stomach. We were down for the count. We simply shook our heads no, and they left.

This is where you learn not to take anything for granted. When Tracey asked, "What kind?" he was not asking for the name. He was asking if the growth was malignant. Because the doctor did not say it was malignant, Tracey assumed he meant the tumor was benign. On the other hand, I knew that oncologist meant CANCER. I had millions of questions but felt that I could not ask them in front of Tracey. I was afraid to ask too many questions—afraid of the answers they would give me. I was not ready to listen to survival statistics. Luckily, all of the new specialists with whom we met were compassionate and did not destroy our hopes with the worst-case scenarios. Tracey needed to live in temporary ignorance of the truth. His understanding was that he was undergoing further treatment as a preventative measure, in order to prevent the tumor from coming back. He was not ready to hear the word "cancer." For the time being it really didn't matter, because "cancer" is only another word. It's how you react that's important.

Tracey was exhausted and fell asleep, but I needed more information. Kost was out of town, and I couldn't remember the names of any of the other doctors who had examined Tracey. I certainly was not going to chance talking to another resident (RULE #3). Luckily, the neurosurgeons' offices were located in the hospital. It was almost 5 P.M. I rushed to the eleventh floor, hoping to catch one of the surgeons. All the physicians were gone, but one of the neuro-oncology nurses talked with me. I wanted to know more but I couldn't articulate my questions. Usually, I am a very direct person and get right to the point. However, my fear made me mute. The nurse talked in generalities. I don't remember much of what she said, except for one statement: "Don't rely on statistics." I made a decision right then that no matter what happened, no matter what we were told, and no matter what I read, Tracey was going to live. Please don't misunderstand me. I was not in a state of denial. I knew that this was serious shit (excuse my language). But, we were going to live our life, and damn the statistics.

The oncologist, Dr. Ira Wollner, visited us first. He was very kind and understood that we were in shock. He gave us a booklet to read regarding brain tumors, overviewed the recommended chemotherapy treatment, suggested that we write down questions, and scheduled an appointment in two weeks. Our brains were on overload; we could only absorb so much.

On Thursday morning, we met the radiation oncologist, Dr. Jae Ho Kim. He asked Tracey to tell him what he knew so far about the diagnosis. Tracey said that he understood that he needed further treatment in order to prevent the tumor from recurring. He couldn't remember the name of the tumor, but he said that it was low grade. Dr. Kim nodded, even though he knew that this was not a low grade tumor. Tracey's attitude was the important thing. He needed hope so that he would have the stamina to fight. Dr. Kim also described the radiation treatment plan and made an appointment for a consultation in three weeks.

By 10:30 A.M., we were going home. Tracey had survived, and we were going home.

Chapter Six

Going Home

We wanted to celebrate Tracey's homecoming, so a few friends came over for dinner. It was a beautiful summer day. We sat out on our deck overlooking the lake and enjoyed Tracey's favorite meal—steaks cooked on the grill and corn on the cob. In the excitement, we forgot that Tracey was still recovering from major surgery. He was exhausted and needed to rest. Everyone excused themselves, and we went to bed at 8 P.M. Tracey was not the only one who was tired. I was asleep before my head hit the pillow. Over the next few days, we received phone calls all through the day and night. Our sleep was constantly interrupted. People cared and wanted to give us their best wishes. But, I was exhausted. I had to do something. So I left a message on the answering machine letting everyone know what time we would answer the phone, and I gave an update on Tracey's condition. This worked really well. Thank God for modern technology.

For the next week, I worked out of our house. Since I was a sales person, I was able to do my phone work at home. I had purchased a laptop computer the previous year, and it was invaluable to me now. All of my account activity and customer phone numbers were readily available, so it wasn't necessary for me to be at the office every day. Sales can be very stressful at times. My life was enough of a roller-coaster without the added pressure of meeting my sales goals. Where my work was concerned, I was very fortunate that the philosophy of my employer, Compuware Corporation, was centered around the importance of family values. Management allowed me the flexibility to come and go as I needed in order to support my husband. Every time a crisis arose, they were always more concerned about my family than they were about the bottom line revenue that I had produced. I have talked to many other families who were not as fortunate. They had to make choices regarding continuing to work and caring for a loved one. Often, there were devastating financial implications in terms of not only paying the bills, but also of being able to maintain insurance coverage. Even though I was not in the office, I was determined to be productive. Compuware's compassion and understanding resulted in my personal determination to exceed their expectations regarding my performance.

I was amazed by Tracey's quick recovery. Within a week, he felt comfortable staying home alone, and I went back to work. Although he wasn't able to drive for at least eight weeks, Tracey was very fortunate. Legally, if he had a seizure, he would not have been able to drive for six months.

His friends made sure that he was not house bound. They called and took him to lunch. One day a buddy picked him up, and they went to the golf course. Tracey was an excellent golfer. Without practicing, he consistently shot in the high 70s for eighteen holes. This particular day, his friend thought he had the advantage. After all, Tracey had just had brain surgery. Tracey beat him by two strokes. His concentration and determination were so strong that he consistently exceeded anyone's expectations of what he should be able to do. This true grit was part of Tracey's character, and it never deserted him.

Since Tracey couldn't do all the active things he enjoyed, he did something he had never done much of before. He watched TV. Up to this time, I had objected to paying for cable TV because we didn't watch many shows. Tracey loved sports and wanted access to the sports shows on ESPN. I agreed. He needed something to occupy his time during the day. It was very difficult for Tracey to be home alone for two reasons. First of all, he enjoyed talking with people. Second, others enjoyed Tracey's company, because his enthusiasm for whatever his interest was contagious. If people visited, he needed to have something interesting that he could discuss. In the long run, two shows other than ESPN became his favorite. The first was the Discovery Channel. He became a nature buff. Not only did he learn many new things about the animal kingdom, but his memory for details and facts was astounding. I was not very interested in TV, but we always watched the Discovery Channel together. The second show that he became addicted to was *Live: Regis & Kathie Lee*. Now this does not seem to make any sense, unless you consider that Tracey really needed to have his spirits lifted. He found the banter between Kathie Lee and Regis entertaining, and it made him laugh. I never understood what made this show so popular until I saw its impact on Tracey. Every day we talked about Regis and Kathie Lee's antics. It was like they were neighbors at whom we could laugh and shake our heads.

Tracey also enjoyed watching videos. He had a small library of ski, golf, and nature videos. I was amazed at how many times he could watch the same videos, sometimes as many as ten times. No matter how many times he watched, he was still fascinated by what he saw. I was not so mesmerized. After I viewed a video once, he had to promise that he would only watch it again when I was not home.

Another way that we passed time was listening to music. Tracey loved lyrics but couldn't carry a tune. I loved melody but didn't pay much attention to the lyrics. I had never really had a favorite song until July 1993, when Tracey was first diagnosed with cancer. For some reason, a song by Sting called "Fields of Gold" caught my attention. The melancholy lyrics tugged at my heart strings. It describes the love of a couple from a man's perspective. He feels that their life together has been a field of gold. He makes a promise that no matter what happens, in the time still left, they will walk in fields of gold. Time passes and he dies. But, he tells his love that things will happen that will give her joy because they will remind her of him. No matter what happens, she should not let her sorrow blind her and prevent her from remembering that, "We walked in fields of gold." Tracey knew why this was my favorite song. I was afraid that I would lose him, and my only comfort would be the memories of our life together. Little did I know that every time he reminded me my favorite song was playing; we were both making the same silent vow—to make sure that in the time still left, we walked in fields of gold.

As he began to feel better, Tracey felt guilty that he was not working. He didn't want to take advantage of me. It was a natural reaction. Men are trained that they are supposed to take care of their families. Because we trusted one another implicitly, we were able to talk about our feelings. Tracey was embarrassed.

He was worried about what other people would think. It was always surprising how thoughtless people could be. One of the frequent questions was, "What about your job? When are you going back to work?" We discussed possible answers and decided on, "My doctors said I shouldn't go back to work yet. My resistance is low, and they want to limit my exposure to viruses." This answer seemed to work.

We were very fortunate because Tracey received three important benefits because of his tenure at Sears & Roebuck Company. The first was that Tracey could take a medical leave of absence for up to one year. This is nine months more than is legally required, and it gave Tracey some job security until he could return to work.

Second, long term medical insurance was affordable. Through Sears' retirement program, the monthly premium was only $75 per month. It included office visits, major medical, and prescription coverage with some deductibles. Most companies only offer insurance during a short term illness. If employees become disabled and are unable to return to work for an extended period of time, they qualify for COBRA rates, which are expensive, for an eighteen month period. Afterwards, there are few guarantees. Social Security benefits may or may not be approved. At this point, many families become financially devastated.

Finally, Sears' short term sick leave policy provided ten weeks of full pay and ten weeks of half pay. This income acted as a buffer until the long term disability insurance, which we had the forethought to purchase, became effective. Even though we were financially stable at this point, we were glad that we had this benefit package. It took the edge off. However, much later we realized that we had underestimated the amount of income we might need if either one us became disabled. We discovered that even though we had good insurance, healthcare costs could easily become astronomical.

I emphasized that his job for the next year was to become healthy. In the meantime, I would continue working. I tried to help Tracey understand that I would work whether he was ill or healthy. It made no difference to me whether Tracey ever worked again. I just wanted him to be healthy. This subject came up every few months. I always reassured him that I loved him. When the time was right, he would work again. Occasionally, other people would complain about having to work. Tracey would always quietly say, "I wish I could work." I silently cried every time he expressed that wish. I always hoped that it would be one of his dreams that would come true.

The effect of Tracey's illness was ironic. Security had always been a major concern. We always made a point of saving a portion of our income. Working was important to both of us. During my first marriage, I quit my job and moved. By the time I was divorced, I had no income, no car, and only $250 in my pocket. I swore that I would never put myself in that position again. I would never allow myself to depend on anyone else financially. Little did I know that one day the tables would be turned, and my family would be financially dependent on me.

Our first return visit to Henry Ford was to remove the eighty staples in Tracey's head. He was worried about the pain. Luckily, I had abdominal surgery ten years previously. I told him not to worry, because it wouldn't hurt. I remember I had been worried but was pleasantly surprised by how quickly and painlessly they were removed. In this case reality was much better than antici-pation. Tracey was relieved when the staple removal was complete with no ill effects.

Tracey's stamina was slowly returning. As the end of August approached, a combination of chemotherapy and radiation were scheduled. Initially, we thought that the surgery had been the major concern. However, we quickly understood that these doctors planned to continue treatment for at least one full year. As a result, we learned more about medicine than we ever wanted or intended to know.

Chapter Seven

Radiation

Four weeks after surgery, Tracey started a combination of radiation and chemotherapy treatments. Before every appointment with his physicians, I wrote down all of our questions and reviewed them with Tracey to see if there was anything else that we wanted to know or clarify. This was a good approach for two reasons. One, we might forget to ask something important; and two, it enabled us to talk about our fears and concerns, which were not always the same. We were still very afraid and in a state of shock. Part of the problem was that we didn't know what questions to ask. We had been given literature to read, but Tracey was not interested. At the time, it upset me that he wasn't taking responsibility for his treatment. What I didn't understand was that he needed me to take some control for him, because he had all he could handle just trying to control his emotions. He needed my help in order to keep a positive attitude.

On the other hand, I couldn't read enough. I called cancer organizations and requested everything that discussed brain tumors and their treatment. The information I received painted a grim picture. A five year survival was considered successful. The statistics were gruesome, but I needed to know the enemy. Tracey did not. I was the strategist, and he was on the front line. No one could possibly do both jobs. He had to have hope. We agreed that statistics did not mean much. He would either survive or he would die. We made a conscious decision to live and enjoy life in the midst of this war.

Up to this point, neither one of us knew anyone who had been diagnosed with a brain tumor. Over the next few months, people came out of the woodwork with stories. For the most part, they were unsolicited and discouraging. I know people were trying to be helpful, so I would listen and then try to forget any doom and gloom forecasts. We didn't need any help getting depressed.

A week before treatment commenced, Tracey began to take high doses of steroids which were intended to reduce brain swelling. Steroids are miracle drugs because without them, radiation would not be possible. However, there are definite side effects, most of which, fortunately, disappear over time. I think that if athletes who try to pump themselves up by using steroids could see the impact of this drug on cancer patients, they would never touch them. Even though athletes consume a different variety of steroid, they do suffer some of the same consequences.

In order to receive radiation and chemotherapy, you must sign a waiver. Potential side effects are listed, and the physician explains the risks. It's a strange feeling to put your trust in the hands of total strangers. You blindly depend on their expertise and hope for the best. Chemotherapy consisted of taking a pill every few days. The purpose was to enhance the effects of radiation. Through techniques that I don't really understand, the radiation oncologist determines the position of the tumor and calculates the required radiation dosage. In Tracey's case, he received three small tattoos (dots) on his scalp. These were used as points of reference for all treatments. Five days a week for seven weeks, he received radiation. The treatments themselves lasted only a couple of minutes. There was no pain, nausea, or discomfort. However, the cumulative effect was that Tracey became very tired and had no energy. Every day at 8 A.M., Monday through Friday, he received radiation. By 11 A.M., he was taking a nap.

It was very important for us to make plans for the future. The previous February, we had arranged to take a water-skiing vacation with five other couples at the end of August. We had rented a houseboat for four days, and we needed to trailer two ski boats and two jet skis from Detroit to the Cumberland Gap in northern Tennessee. Tracey's physicians encouraged us to go. After a week of radiation, we drove nine hours and met our friends. Even though Tracey couldn't water-ski, it was a wonderful escape. We relaxed, laughed, and revitalized ourselves. A change of scenery was exactly what we needed. I know some people thought we were crazy, but we were determined to enjoy ourselves. We were not going to stop living.

By the end of the third week of treatment, Tracey started to have reactions to the steroids. He became short-tempered and was restless at night. The muscles in his legs were deteriorating. In addition, he had intermittent joint pain that was so severe that he could barely walk. Fortunately, if he took anti-inflammatory medication, such as Advil, this arthritis-like pain was relieved.

The first time he experienced severe pain in his joints, Tracey looked like an old man trying to walk. Needless to say, I was very concerned because we had not been informed that this was a side effect from the steroids. For all we knew, it could be a result of the surgery or—worse yet—a recurrence of the tumor. A friend was taking him for his radiation treatment, and Tracey planned to talk with the radiation oncologist who was on call. By 10 A.M., I had not heard from Tracey. I was worried and impatient. What had the doctor said? I tried to call Tracey, but all the phones in our neighborhood were out of order. I called the doctor. Blood had been drawn, and the results did not show anything out of the ordinary. Tracey had been told to go home and rest. By 2 P.M., I was frantic because I still couldn't reach Tracey. I raced home, but he was not there. Where could he be? Just as I got home, our friend, Jennifer, came to the house to check on Tracey. I was getting ready to call emergency rooms. As Jennifer was leaving, Tracey came home with his sister, Claudia. Jennifer looked at Tracey and said, "I hope that those aren't golf clubs that I see on your shoulder." Tracey knew he was in trouble. I was furious. Claudia excused herself because she could see the atomic mushroom cloud over my head and was afraid of the fallout. This was the straw that broke the camel's back. I had had enough. Tracey and I needed to sit down and talk.

For a couple of weeks, Tracey had refused to read any information about his tumor and had been telling everyone that it was benign. No doctor had said the word "cancer" yet. I had been trying to remain sympathetic. He was in a state of denial. But, I felt that he had gone too far. The doctor had told him to rest. Because he felt better, he decided that he needed to push himself physically. We needed a reality check. I asked him what he knew about his tumor. He was convinced that it was benign. I then broke the news that it was malignant. His face dropped and

I'll never forget his next question, "Are you telling me that I am going to die?" I told him, "No, what I'm telling you is that we have a battle ahead, and you need to listen to the doctors." He became defensive and said, "Well, I'm not going to stop doing the things that I enjoy doing. Besides, the physician I saw was not my doctor. I don't like him." I agreed with him that he shouldn't have to give up the things he liked to do. However, in fairness to me, since what he did impacted my life too, he should not totally ignore advice until he checked with a physician he respected and trusted. It was our first post-operative fight. There would be other arguments, but they were amazingly few and far between. For the most part, they arose when we became self-absorbed and were not sensitive enough to each other's needs.

At the beginning of October 1993, we had an eight week follow-up visit with Kost, Tracey's neurosurgeon. By this time, we had had a chance to digest information, and we asked many questions. Not only did Kost help us understand the nature of the tumor, but he was concerned about our emotional well-being as a couple. He asked us how we were getting along. With a chagrined look, I said that we had fought that morning. Tracey wanted to be pampered, and I was willing to cooperate up to a point. He was very vain about his hair, and I frequently joked that Tracey needed three hours to get ready to go anywhere. Of that time, two hours were spent styling his hair. Now his hair was falling out in clumps, and he was bald except for a strip about four inches wide down the center of his head. That particular morning, he decided that he wanted me to blow dry and comb his hair because he couldn't do anything with it. This does not seem like an unreasonable request, except that I felt overwhelmed. I was responsible for practically everything, and Tracey was beginning to take advantage of me by acting helpless. When I refused to style his hair, he was angry. I was at the end of my rope; I yelled, "I can't do everything!" I stomped into the bedroom and began sobbing. Tracey knew he had crossed the line but pretended that nothing had happened. His way of apologizing was to pay me a compliment. Unfortunately, he chose to admire my hairstyle. I thought he was being sarcastic. My eyes widened, my forehead became furrowed, and my right eyebrow went up. When my right eyebrow goes up, watch out; it's a sure sign of trouble for anyone within twenty-five feet. My stare would have stopped a raging grizzly bear in its tracks. At that moment, we had the good sense to call a truce. Then, Tracey came up with a solution to his dilemma; he'd get a haircut.

Understandably, it really bothered Tracey that he might have a mohawk hairdo for the rest of his life. But he was willing to endure practically anything, if it meant that he would survive. Kost suggested that Tracey take Vitamin E pills and massage his scalp with Vitamin E cream. In about four months, Tracey once again had a full head of hair. Unfortunately, he renewed his driver's license when he looked like a very bloated Ernie (of Muppet fame). Months later, a bank teller asked for a picture ID. Tracey handed over his driver's license. The teller looked back and forth between Tracey and his ID a few times, grinned and said, "Nice do!" I tried to persuade Tracey to get another picture taken for his license, but he ignored me. I think his driver's license was his badge of courage. It was proof of how far he had come.

Hair loss, combined with the bloating caused by steroids, really affects a patient's self-esteem. By October 1993, Tracey's appearance had changed so drastically that friends who had known him for twenty years did not recognize him. As he approached the end of radiation, he looked and felt exhausted. Depression hit him like a sledge hammer. I became very concerned, because he was withdrawing into himself, again. His sense of humor disappeared. We tried to celebrate when radiation was complete, but Tracey had less energy and enthusiasm than I had ever seen in him. The only real pleasure he experienced at this time was his last day of radiation. Naomi and Sally, the radiation technicians, had become his friends. They called him their buddy and presented him with a graduation diploma. I had almost forgotten how the simplest things people do for one another are often the gifts that mean the most. I'm not sure why, but Tracey received many gifts. Perhaps it was because he expected nothing, but he appreciated every gift that was offered.

I tried to entice him with his favorite foods. Since nothing tasted very good, he lost his appetite. I tried to pamper him, but he didn't want to be touched. I was worried. In two weeks, Dr. Wollner wanted to start yet another protocol of chemotherapy. Where was Tracey going to find the strength to withstand the onslaught of poisonous drugs?

Chapter Eight

Chemotherapy

We hoped that two weeks was enough of a break. Tracey was very tired, but he didn't want to postpone his first treatment. Dr. Wollner had emphasized the importance of beginning as soon as possible. Tracey was apprehensive. No one ever had a good story to tell about chemotherapy. Movies and television programs added to the unspoken fear of all patients and their families. Dr. Wollner tried to reassure us that the side effects would be minimal, "Most people do not experience any nausea. Fatigue is probably the most likely side effect." He gave us literature describing symptoms to report and foods to avoid, such as chocolate, aged cheese, and red wine. Most people don't realize there are many types of drugs that physicians prescribe for different types of cancers. There is also more than one protocol, or regimen of treatment, which can be recommended for a specific cancer. In Tracey's case, the recommended chemotherapy protocol was called PCV. It was a combination of drugs, some of which would be administered intravenously on an outpatient basis, while others would be taken orally at home. This cycle would be repeated every twenty-eight days for the next year. I thought this was ironic as a treatment plan for a man, considering women learn to count twenty-eight days early in life. We were given a calendar (does this sound familiar ladies?) so we could keep track of Tracey's medication. It was very confusing. In order to reduce the risk of administering drugs incorrectly, Tracey relied on my help. Since he took all pills with meals and at bedtime, I purchased four containers. Each was a different color and I labeled them "breakfast," "lunch," "dinner," and "bed." This was a simple way to ensure that he took the right pills at the correct times.

The first day of chemotherapy, Tracey needed to go to the clinic. We made an early morning appointment, because he didn't want to wait all day. Tracey may have been afraid of chemotherapy, but he was petrified of needles. A blood sample had to be drawn. This was a weekly ritual, because the doctors needed to track the impact of the drugs. They didn't want his cell counts to go too low. They were trying to kill the cancer, not Tracey. Unfortunately, chemo has a tendency not to distinguish between the patient and the disease.

Once the IV had been started, the nurses invited me to keep Tracey company. They were waiting for the results from the bloodwork before beginning. The nurses were very good and had explained everything that would happen. Well, almost everything. There is always the unexpected. Tracey was very anxious and his right foot was twitching a mile a minute. He whispered, "I feel funny." Without another word, Tracey became very pale, his eyes rolled back in his head, and he passed out. Within a few moments, a cardiologist, a neurologist, and three nurses were in the room. It was a doctor's worst nightmare. A few minutes later, Tracey regained consciousness. Apparently, all the needles made him lightheaded. They gave him fruit juice and were able to proceed without any further problems. We went home, and Tracey had a snack but was afraid to eat much of anything. He didn't want to get sick. The rest of the day was uneventful.

The next day at noon, Tracey needed to take a pill, Procarbazine. We thought that if he coated his stomach with yogurt, it might reduce the chances of nausea. Other than being very tired, he was fine until about 2 P.M. Suddenly, he ran upstairs to the bathroom and vomited for the next two hours. I tried giving him nausea medication, ginger ale, ice cream, and tea. Nothing stayed down, and he was becoming dehydrated. I called Dr. Wollner. Within a couple of minutes, he was on the phone. He couldn't understand why Tracey was so sick. He kept saying, "I've never seen this reaction." He wanted to admit him to the hospital, but Tracey wouldn't agree. Finally, I made him promise to go to Emergency if he wasn't better in two hours. As long as he didn't try to eat or drink anything, he was okay. By the next morning, he was still a little bit queasy, but could drink fluids. He looked totally drained. I was applying a cold compress to his forehead and he whispered, "I can't do this anymore." My mind said, "If you don't keep trying, you'll die." But my heart cried, "You're right. No one understands why you have been so sick. But you can only do what you can do." Although Tracey had just begun the first cycle of chemotherapy, it was time to stop.

Tracey did not like confrontation, and would defer problems to me. I told him if he decided to stop chemo, that was fine with me, however, he had to be the one to call the doctor. I would not do it. I felt that Tracey needed to take control of his life, and this would be the first step. Dr. Wollner graciously accepted Tracey's decision. Immediately afterward, Tracey's whole mental attitude changed. It was amazing. He started smiling and telling jokes. The man I knew was coming back. He was able to look to the future. He had dignity again.

Since Tracey was stable and did not experience any further reactions, I resumed my normal work schedule. I know that Tracey was distressed when I needed to leave town on business trips, but he never complained. In fact, he encouraged me to travel and enjoyed my success. It was the closest he could come to working. He gave me advice, and almost every day he asked if I sold anything. He knew my accounts and many of my customers' names. I jokingly told my boss that I didn't need a manager at work because I had one at home. I needed to continue working not only for financial reasons, but also for my mental health. I could not live Tracey's illness twenty-four hours a day. Work was my temporary escape.

After Thanksgiving, we had a follow-up visit with Dr. Eleanor Walker, a radiation oncologist. Tracey calmly broke the news that he had stopped chemo, at which point I began to cry. I couldn't hold back the floodgates. My feelings of frustration and fear poured out with my tears. Dr. Walker talked with us and listened to our horrible experience. She understood why Tracey had made his decision, and told us, "Take some time and enjoy the holidays. You need a break."

It was our favorite season. Tracey had the energy to visit friends, and he was enjoying himself for the first time in five months. A sense of peace was returning to our lives as we celebrated Christmas with Shelley. We weren't interested in a lot of excitement. Quiet time with our family was what we needed.

In January 1994, Tracey was confined to the house because the weather was freezing cold. He needed a change of scenery and climate. His parents lived in Florida. It was a perfect place for him to recuperate. For three weeks, he enjoyed the warm temperatures and sunshine. While Tracey was in Florida, I received a call from the neuro-oncology department at Henry Ford. A neurologist, Dr. Tom Mikkelsen, wanted to make an appointment to discuss an alternative chemotherapy protocol. As long as the nausea could be controlled, I knew that I could convince Tracey to reconsider treatment. I scheduled a time to meet during the first week of February. I would tell Tracey when he returned to Michigan. Right now, he needed to rest, relax, and enjoy himself.

I was relieved that Tracey's physicians had not forgotten him. They knew that no drug would be effective unless Tracey's spirit had a chance to heal. Since so many medical disciplines are involved in treating patients with brain cancer, a brain tumor board had been created. In this way, individual cases could be discussed and each patient's treatment plan monitored and planned through a team approach. We had a neurosurgeon, a radiation oncologist, an oncologist, and now a neurologist. Each had his own focus. It was important to have a central contact not only to keep track of Tracey's progress but also to be available if we had questions. Tom Mikkelsen became this lifeline for us. We were very lucky, because we were always treated as individuals rather than as a car on an assembly line.

After he returned from Florida, Tracey agreed to listen to what his doctors had in mind. When we arrived for our appointment, we were escorted to a waiting room. After a few minutes, the door opened and Tom Mikkelsen walked in. Remember first impressions. Well, my first thought was, "Does Henry Ford Hospital recruit its doctors from the Doogie Howser School of Medicine?" Tom was very sympathetic and profes-sional, and he looked very young. In addition to reviewing Tracey's medical background and treatment, he spent time getting to know us. After we discussed an alternative chemo protocol and the precautions that would be taken to prevent nausea, Tracey agreed to, "Give it another shot." Tom quickly called Ira Wollner (was this prearranged?) and sent us off to meet with him. They were not going to take any chances and allow Tracey an opportunity to change his mind. If they had their way, Tracey would have started immediately. However, Tracey took control and agreed to begin in three days. He wanted to enjoy the weekend.

The new treatment was called BCNU. It was administered intravenously at a clinic on an outpatient basis over three consecutive days. Each treatment lasted about three hours and a six week rest period followed. The same cycle would be repeated six additional times—as long as there was not a recurrence of a tumor. We had a year of chemotherapy to count down.

Before each treatment, Tracey received an intravenous dose of nausea medication called Zofran. As a precaution, he also took Zofran orally for a few days. Fortunately, Tracey tolerated the first cycle well. Nevertheless, he was very tired and his energy level was low until it was time to start the next cycle. Since the drugs themselves could be lethal if they were not administered correctly, it was essential to test his blood on a weekly basis. Every six weeks, we met with Dr. Wollner in preparation for the next cycle. We had to wait and see if there were any other side effects.

For some reason, Tracey did not experience any hair loss. Outwardly, he looked healthy. Most people would have been unable to tell that he was fighting brain cancer. This had good and bad points. On the one hand, people did not avoid Tracey, because he didn't act or look sick. On the other hand, friends were not always sensitive. Even though Tracey looked normal, he needed to be very structured regarding eating meals, resting during the day, limiting physical activity, and avoiding people with colds. We were structured not because we wanted to be, but in order to protect Tracey's health, we had to be less flexible.

An aggravating problem arose. The veins in Tracey's arms were scarred from the chemo. It was becoming more and more difficult for the nurses to find a good vein. Occasionally, a technician would poke him three times. He complained, and I told him to take control. He needed to speak up and request someone else. If someone had a problem drawing blood, the rule of thumb became, "More than one poke and you're out." This might seem a little harsh, but if you were poked with a needle more than fifty-two times in one year, your tolerance would be low too. One day, Tracey watched a trainee try three times to draw blood from another patient. As the trainee approached, Tracey told her to go get someone else because she wasn't going to practice on him. She was irritated, but I was proud. Patients can easily become victims, but Tracey would not succumb. He was finally taking some control. Of course, it helped to have me standing behind him for moral support and for the occasional push in the right direction.

Before we knew it, five months had passed. It was the Fourth of July, 1994, and we were going to have a party. It had become an annual event that our friends looked forward to celebrating. During the early part of the day, Tracey and I were getting the house ready for company. The house was clean, the food was prepared, the flowers were planted, and the grass was mowed. The only thing left to do was weedwhack. Every year I bought a new weedwhacker because we purchased inexpensive electric models. That year, I decided to spend a little more money and bought a deluxe gas model. It was a little temperamental, and I felt a little awkward as I was trying to start it. When I pulled on the cord for the third time, I realized why I was having difficulty. For some reason, I was using my left arm instead of my right. You see, I am right handed. But more importantly, I was in excruciating pain. The pulling motion caused my left shoulder to dislocate, and to say I was screaming is an understatement. There is a famous scene in the movie *Lethal Weapon 2* where Mel Gibson slams his dislocated shoulder into a wall in order to pop it back in place, but no, this is not what I did. I might have been in pain, but I was not stupid or crazy. Fortunately, it was a subluxation instead of a total dislocation. By sheer luck, I sat up straight, dropped my arm, and my shoulder slid back into place. This sounds simple. Unfortunately, my summer plans were ruined. All the things that I loved to do, such as golf, tennis, and water-skiing were out of the question. At first, Tracey was worried. When he realized that I was all right, he started to reprimand me for trying to start the weedwhacker. When he saw my raised eyebrow, he had enough sense to change tactics. He tried to make me feel better, but he didn't have much success. I was sobbing not because I was in pain, but because I was totally depressed. Finally, I told him, "Just leave me alone. I'll be okay. I just need time to feel sorry for myself." I know he was thinking, "I hope this doesn't take long because we have company coming in three hours." I finished crying and decided I could choose either to be happy or to be depressed. In either case, I would still have an injured shoulder. That fact would not change. I know everyone was amazed, but I actually had a good time that day. We barbecued hamburgers, lounged in the hot tub, watched the fireworks display, and enjoyed the holiday with our friends and family.

In mid July 1994, Tracey was scheduled for a CAT scan. It had been a year since surgery and six months since the last scan. I was no longer confident about test results. We were both gun-shy. I agreed to call for the results, because Tracey was too nervous. I remember holding my breath as I waited for Dr. Wollner to say, "Everything looks good." It was like winning the lottery. I placed the phone in its cradle and burst into tears. I was almost hyperventilating. At the time, I was in my office, and two co-workers heard my sobs. They were afraid to ask me what was wrong. They weren't sure what to do. They simply came in and gave me a hug. It was the first of many hugs that I received from co-workers and friends when words of joy or sorrow were impossible.

I collected myself and dialed our home phone number. Tracey answered, and I burst out with the great news. I waited for a scream of joy but only heard silence. This was not the reaction I had anticipated. I was confused. Wasn't he excited? I'm not sure why I expected uncontrolled screams when I had been speechless. I realized that we didn't have the luxury of letting down our defenses. Tracey had won a skirmish, but had not yet won the war. He had three more treatments before he was home free. Thanksgiving would be time enough to celebrate.

In the meantime, we were going to enjoy the summer.

Chapter Nine

Merry Christmas and Have a Happy New Year

We celebrated Thanksgiving quietly. Tracey had just completed his last chemo treatment. I was relieved that it was finally over. Sally, the nurse who administered Tracey's treatments, took his picture and placed it in the clinic hall of fame. His graduation present was a bottle of sparkling cider. My cousin, Barb, planned a small family celebration. Tracey deserved recognition for what he had achieved.

Even though Tracey looked healthy, I was still holding my breath. We were emotionally high, but physically we were both burned out. We needed a chance to refuel our energy. As I expected, Tracey started to worry about going back to work. I told him that he needed to rest. Work could wait until March. Physically, he couldn't possibly be ready until then.

We decided to go to Florida for Christmas. Tracey flew to Ft. Myers to visit his parents. I joined him a week later. After exchanging gifts, we were going to visit my uncle and aunt before heading to Clearwater to see my folks. As we approached my uncle and aunt's condominium, Tracey asked me to stop the car. He had something to tell me. I shifted into park and turned off the ignition. We really hadn't had a chance to embrace. After all, it had been over a week since we had seen one another. I briefly thought, "How romantic!"—until I saw his eyes brimming with tears. I slipped off my seat belt, put my arms around him and asked, "What's wrong?" The previous morning he had experienced new symptoms. The left side of his face and his left fingers had gone temporarily numb. It had happened once and lasted only five minutes, but we were both crying. We were scared. We gathered up all the courage we could muster, put smiles on our faces, and truly enjoyed our Christmas vacation. We were both afraid that it would be the last Christmas that we would spend together. We were determined to enjoy ourselves, and we did. We walked on the beach, played a little golf, and loved one another. Our gifts to one another were centered on the sport that we loved the most. I received new snow skis and boots; Tracey received a new HellyHansen ski outfit, which was specially designed for deep powder skiing. We had planned a family ski vacation to the Whistler/Blackcomb resort in Vancouver, Canada, at the end of February, to celebrate Shelley's twenty-first birthday. Additionally, Tracey was going to have a dream come true. He was going to go helicopter skiing.

Every year we always exchanged ornaments that had some personal meaning. Not only was our Christmas tree beautiful, but it represented memories of our life together. Tracey always gave me a Waterford crystal ornament which was part of a series called the "Twelve Days of Christmas." This year was Eleven Pipers Piping. Even though I knew what he was giving me, I could hardly wait to add the newest piece to the collection. The next gift was an unspoken tradition. Tracey knew that I loved Christmas music, and he added to my collection every year. He had been listening to the radio, and a song by Mariah Carey caught his attention. He told me that this was his favorite Christmas carol. I loved the melody but couldn't pay close attention to the lyrics because its title was "I'll Miss You Most at Christmas." Tracey and I were sending messages back and forth to one another through music. We couldn't bear to talk about the possibility of his death with one another, because then it would become a reality. Music was the way that we could let each other know what we were feeling.

We told no one about the new symptoms. There wasn't anything that anybody could do. The symptoms had disappeared. Maybe it was nothing. Tracey was scheduled to have a CAT scan during the second week of January. As long as nothing changed, we would call our doctors when we got home to Detroit.

Since Dr. Wollner was the last physician we had seen, I called him. As long as the symptoms had not recurred, he said not to worry and to wait for the CAT scan that was scheduled for the following week.

I never traveled when Tracey had tests. I had learned my lesson. However, the day we expected the results, I was participating in a major client presentation that lasted all day. During a break, I called Dr. Wollner from a phone booth. He was paged. He had reviewed the results and had just talked with Tracey. I held my breath until he said, "I'm sorry to tell you this, Kathy, but it seems that Tracey has a recurrence." He didn't have the details. As soon as I hung up the receiver, I called home. Tracey was not outwardly upset. He was numb. He told me not to worry and to go back to my meeting. I was getting a lot of experience putting on a poker face. It was almost like I had multiple personalities, because I was able to hide my grief and anxiety from most people. I had the ability to put myself into autopilot. It was my mechanism for handling what needed to be done. Luckily, I only had to socialize with customers for a short period of time. I'm sure that no one realized that I felt like my world was falling apart.

We needed to talk with Tom Mikkelsen, our neurologist, in order to get a recommendation for further treatment. Tom arranged to have a joint appointment that included Kost. On Wednesday, January 25, 1995, we met with Tom and Kost. The results were not encouraging. The tumor had reappeared in the same area, the right frontal lobe of the brain, but was larger than the original growth. It was three centimeters, which is about the size of an egg. It had invaded some motor control areas. The good news was that it was operable, and Kost said he could operate the following week. There was a different chemotherapy protocol which would follow. Since BCNU had not stopped the tumor from growing, a different chemo protocol was recommended. We had been thinking about getting a second opinion. Now we were sure that we wanted a second opinion. Since we lived in a major metropolitan area, we were able to find another specialist who agreed to see us on short notice. It was scheduled for that afternoon. Tom arranged to have copies of Tracey's records and CAT scan available for us. We needed a medical case history for our next meeting.

We arrived for our appointment, and a nurse explained that a resident would do the initial examination. Then the neurosurgeon would meet with us. The resident was very thorough. He read the medical records and viewed the scans. He began testing Tracey's reflexes, strength, balance, senses, and memory. Tracey had just begun to have dexterity problems with his left fingers, and his gait on the left side had changed. As the exam continued, I could tell that Tracey had lost some sensation on the left side as well. The resident took notes and then disappeared. In a few minutes, the neurosurgeon came in the room with the resident, the nurse, and two other doctors (interns). He asked a few questions and began testing Tracey's reflexes. Tracey and I began to feel uncomfortable. We both felt like Tracey was a bug on a slide being inspected, poked, and prodded. Knowing glances were passed from doctor to doctor. It was as if we weren't supposed to know or couldn't possibly understand the significance of the tests that were being performed. We were being treated like we were stupid. We weren't stupid. We were afraid. I understand that medical rounds are important, for how else can doctors learn? However, these doctors were learning very poor communication skills. They were learning to communicate bad news without saying a word. We were there to find out if their recommendation was the same as the one we had received at Henry Ford. I told them what had been recommended. They said surgery was necessary, but only fifty percent of the tumor could be removed. Otherwise, Tracey would lose total use of his left side. The intermittent numbness Tracey had experienced could have been a seizure. Dilantin, a drug that prevents seizures, was strongly recommended. The choice of chemotherapy was different, but when I asked the neurosurgeon the reason for this particular protocol, he became defensive and authoritative. He acted like I didn't have the right to question his choice. I was simply asking for more information so that we could make an informed decision. In a clipped tone, he said, "I have done research and written papers, and this is what I recommend." Even though he was cordial and asked us if we had any more questions, his actions spoke louder than words. We would not ask him any more questions. We had the information that we needed. We already had doctors whom we trusted and who were willing to listen and answer our questions without becoming defensive.

We called and left a message for Tom that we wanted to schedule the surgery. However, we had questions regarding the chemotherapy recommendation. The next day Tom called back and explained that he had suggested a protocol that did not include Procarbazine, the drug which had made Tracey so ill. Procarbazine was his first choice. However, Tracey needed to continue with chemo, and he didn't want to take any chances that Tracey would give up. Surgery was scheduled for Friday, February 3, at 1 P.M. We would make a decision regarding chemo later.

We also discussed the need for seizure medication. Since seizures are a frequent symptom of brain tumors, Tom and Kost were not sure why Tracey had not experienced this problem. In most cases, Dilantin probably would have been prescribed immediately after the initial diagnosis. However, one of Kost's specialties was treating seizure patients. Based on his knowledge and expertise, he did not feel Dilantin was initially necessary. Why medicate if there is not a problem? Tracey and I wholeheartedly agreed with this philosophy. However, because of this tumor recurrence, it was a matter of time before seizures would occur. They both felt that it was time to prescribe Dilantin. We were not overly concerned, but you always need to be aware of the side effects. One more drug was being added to the mix. In order to monitor the levels of the drug, Tracey would need to have his blood tested occasionally. This is another example of how Tracey was treated as an individual rather than just another patient. There were no cookie cutter treatments: you have a brain tumor so this is what we will do. There were no easy answers, but we always felt that we were included in the decision making process, and therefore, we were ultimately in control. Tracey knew he had doctors who cared about him as a person. He trusted them.

Although his Friday appointment was only a week away, it felt like an eternity. I decided that we couldn't just wait around doing nothing. There was snow on the ground, so we were going to go away for a couple of days and ski in northern Michigan. It wasn't helicopter skiing out West, but Tracey wore his new HellyHansen outfit. He was having more difficulty walking, but I decided if he killed himself skiing, at least he would die happy. We arrived at Boyne Mountain and bought our lift tickets. Tracey couldn't walk and carry his equipment at the same time, so I made a couple of trips to the car, helped him buckle his boots, and carried his skis to the lift line. As we were standing in line for the chairlift, Tracey dropped his ski pole twice. He was losing the ability to grip the handle. This might seem dangerous, but Tracey was an expert skier. I was a much better skier than when we had met, but I would never ski at Tracey's level of expertise. Nonetheless, my competitive nature, which was just as strong as Tracey's, never gave up hope. This was my chance if there ever was one. I might be able to beat him skiing to the bottom of the hill because his strength was limited and his endurance was low. I secured our boot buckles at the top of the hill, and we took off. It was like Tracey was on wings. Even though he wasn't as aggressive as usual, I was unable to reach the bottom of the hill first. It was much closer than ever before, but he still beat me. I hadn't told Tracey what I was up to, because after all, I wanted to have as much of an advantage as I could. When we were sitting in the chair lift, he asked me how he looked skiing down the hill. At this point, I had to tell him what I had tried to do. We laughed and then just enjoyed skiing together for the next two days.

When Friday finally arrived, surgery seemed less intimidating. We knew what to expect, or so we thought. Since we didn't need to be at the hospital until 11 A.M., Shelley met us at admitting. Tracey had opted to shave his head. This time there would be no small bag of hair. I kissed him and then rubbed his bald head for good luck. It would be a very long day. Because of scheduling problems, surgery was delayed and did not begin until practically 3 P.M. The nurse also explained that Kost had performed a five hour surgery that morning. He had squeezed Tracey in because he didn't want him to have to wait another week. I was amazed. Where did Kost get his energy? His compassion was remarkable. For some reason, we were unbelievably lucky. I'm not sure how many were involved, but I was beyond grateful to all the people who worked late that Friday in order to care for Tracey.

Tracey's parents were arriving from Florida that evening. Friends and family wanted to be with us during the surgery, but I told them not to come. If I needed anything, my cousin Jake, who worked at Henry Ford Hospital, would be available. I did not have the patience or energy to talk with anyone other than Shelley. I was not in the mood for idle conversation. We received a progress report during surgery. Everything was okay. At 5 P.M., a friend, Colleen, unexpectedly arrived in the waiting room, and we decided to have dinner in the cafeteria. I wasn't sure if I wanted company. I didn't want sympathy. I didn't want anyone to hold my hand. I just wanted this surgery to be over. Colleen has a very good sense of humor and was able to distract Shelley and me with her stories. The next two hours went by in what seemed like a snap of the fingers. Jake appeared in the waiting room. Surgery was successful, and Kost would talk with us in a few minutes. I was relieved.

We were the last people in the surgical waiting room. As Kost approached us, I grasped his hand and thanked him for his help.

He had very deep circles under his eyes. He did not look so young tonight. Something was wrong. He escorted us to a small room, and before we had a chance to sit down he said, "I had to hurt Tracey." He had our attention. What did he mean? Kost explained that he had been able to remove all visible signs of the tumor. As a result, the side of Tracey's face would droop and he would experience some weakness on his left side. I remember thinking, "That's not so bad. At least he was able to remove the tumor. Tracey had a better chance to survive. I would not lose my best friend, my soul mate." Kost had my undivided attention. My eyes were locked on his. What I saw was hope and determination, not despair and defeat. His final words were, "Tracey has to fight." I didn't say anything, but my internal reaction was, "Well of course Tracey will fight! There is no other choice! We are going to win this battle." As he left, I shook his hand and said, "It's been a long day, Kost. Thank you for your help." He looked at me thoughtfully for a second, and with a tired smile said, "You're welcome."

Now, my attention turned to Shelley. She was crying. Her dad might not be able to do the things that he loved to do. People hear and react differently to the same information. Shelley needed reassurance. I was excited because I thought that Kost would only be able to remove fifty percent of the tumor. He had been able to do much more than I expected. Tracey's chances for survival were better. I explained this to Shelley, and it seemed like she felt a little better. I reminded her that her dad had miraculously recovered from polio as a child. He would recover from this surgery too. He just needed our support. It had been a very long day, and we probably would not be able to see Tracey for three or four hours. Shelley needed to go home and get some rest. I told her to leave and to come back tomorrow. I would stay until I was sure that Tracey was okay.

At 9 P.M., the receptionist told me that Tracey had been moved to intensive care. I could see him. Since it was evening, Tracey was moved from recovery sooner. When I walked into the ICU, he was more alert than after the first surgery. He was afraid that I had deserted him, for he had been in intensive care for an hour. Where had I been? I was his anchor, and he did not feel safe unless he could see and touch me. I looked at his face, but it looked fine. Where was the droop that Kost described? Tracey was afraid. He couldn't move his left side. I explained that there would be some weakness, but his strength would come back. It would just take time. He drifted off to sleep. The nurses awakened him and asked the same questions as before, but this time Tracey did not tell any jokes. At 11 P.M., the nurse told me to go home and get some rest. Tracey was stable, but I was reluctant to leave. Finally, common sense took hold and I realized that I needed sleep. I kissed Tracey goodnight. I would be back tomorrow morning.

When I arrived at 9 A.M. on Saturday, I acted confident and walked into ICU before visiting hours began. I also brought a bribe—donuts. Food is always a good distraction and opens many doors that might otherwise be closed. Tracey could never drink enough coffee, so I bought him a cup of a specialty blend. He was glad to see me. He was sitting in a chair but was subdued. Eating breakfast was difficult because Tracey could not use both hands. It's amazing how many things that we take for granted require two hands—buttering toast, cutting meat, tearing a salt packet, and opening juice containers. Over the next week, the food trays were frequently set down on tables which Tracey couldn't reach without help. I realized that someone needed to be there during meals, because staffing at the hospital was limited. It was going to be hard enough to keep Tracey's spirits up without this kind of added frustration.

I inspected his face. Where was this droop that Kost described? Tracey still didn't have the ability to move his left arm and leg. He was worried. I tried to reassure him, but I was concerned too. This was more than weakness. Tracey motioned for me to come close. He had a story to tell, but this one was not funny. During the night, the patient directly across from Tracey had died. The drapes had been drawn so Tracey could not see much, but he heard everything. Everyone knows that healthcare professionals need to stay detached so they can survive the inevitable death of some patients. However, Tracey saw their eyes and heard their whispered words. He knew that they were in pain. Even though he was worried about his own mortality, he was also concerned about his caregivers. This sensitivity was part of Tracey's character, and it grew as time went by.

Before I left the house, I talked to Tracey's family and told them the results of surgery. His father and sister came to visit. I didn't want to tire Tracey, so I left and went to the waiting room. Within fifteen minutes, Tracey wanted me. Our relationship changed on this day. I became the only person he fully trusted. It was a heavy responsibility, but I would have done anything for him and expected nothing in return. It was a different kind of love. It cannot be explained. It can only be felt.

Shelley visited with Tracey for awhile, but he frequently dozed. For most of the day, I tried to stay in the waiting room. He needed to rest, and I told him that I would be near. If he needed me, he could call for me. The day passed by very slowly. He would not be moved to Step Down until after he had a CAT scan on Sunday. At about 8 P.M., I went home and fell into an exhausted sleep.

The next morning, Tracey could move his toes. It was good news, but I was still worried. We wouldn't be able to talk with Kost or Tom until Monday. I didn't understand why there was this much so-called weakness. About 10 A.M., Dr. Cauliflower (I can't remember his real name) introduced himself. He had assisted Kost during the surgery. Did we have any questions? We talked in generalities for a few minutes and then he excused himself. He had other patients in the ICU on whom he needed to check. The nurse announced that an escort would be taking Tracey for his CAT scan. They needed to get him ready.

I took this opportunity to excuse myself and approach Dr. Cauliflower. Did he have a minute to talk with me? Now, you have to realize that I was having a temporary lapse of memory, and Dr. Cauliflower had done a very good job of camouflaging his true identity. Dr. Cauliflower was a resident, and I had forgotten the most important rule of all, RULE #3—NEVER TALK TO A RESIDENT! He was very courteous and volunteered to sit in a private area and talk. I didn't think that it would take very long. I had a quick question that would only take a minute. I explained that I was concerned about Tracey. Kost had said that there would be weakness, but Tracey couldn't move his left side. Was anything wrong? His eyes brightened, and then he proceeded to dig a hole so deep that most people would have required a backhoe. As we were standing over a trash bin about thirty feet from Tracey, he proceeded to tell me that they were just trying to make Tracey comfortable. He would be able to raise his left shoulder but would never be able to use his left hand again. I was speechless. I was coming to the realization that we would not just be postponing our ski vacation to Whistler/Blackcomb. Tracey would never be able to water-ski, play golf, or snow ski again. Dr. Cauliflower couldn't stop talking. He had diarrhea of the mouth. He explained that Tracey's tumor had changed from an astrocytoma to a glioblastoma, a much more aggressive type of cancer. I was shocked. This was an entirely new diagnosis. How could he be saying this? The pathology report hadn't been completed yet. He realized his error and changed the subject.

Unfortunately, he kept on digging. He said that astrocytoma tumors scared him. I wanted to scream. For God's sake, he was the doctor. Why was he telling me he was scared? He finished his prognosis by telling me that Tracey only had one year, maybe two, to live. Tears were running down my face. Just then I realized that the drapes had been pulled back, and Tracey could clearly see that I was crying. I was leaning on the garbage can and felt like I was going to throw up. Maybe my aim would be good and I'd hit Dr. Cauliflower squarely in the chest. I excused myself from Dr. Cauliflower's clutches, turned, took a deep breath, and walked back to Tracey. He asked me what was wrong. I sighed and said I was just tired. I wasn't very convincing, but Tracey knew me well enough. My lips were sealed. Just then, Dr. Cauliflower caught my eyes. He had what I call The Look. There are no words with The Look, only sympathy and sorrow. At that moment, I had to look away or I would have exploded in anger. I felt like I was part of a horror movie; I felt like Dr. Cauliflower had just slammed me against the wall. It seemed as if every time I tried to move, he drove another stake into my chest. We needed to leave ICU before he could wreak any more havoc in our lives.

Just then Shelley arrived, and we all walked to the basement of the hospital for Tracey's CAT scan. Tracey quizzed Shelley, "Has Kathy said anything to you? Is there something that I'm not being told?" Fortunately, Shelley was in the dark too. She didn't have any new information.

This was one of the darkest times during Tracey's illness. His enthusiasm for life was centered around physical activity. He once mentioned to me that if he couldn't do the things he loved, he would not want to live. In one brief conversation, this resident had almost robbed Tracey of his strongest weapon in his fight against cancer: HOPE. Suddenly, I was pissed. How dare he? I had a choice, and that choice was to believe that Tracey would beat the odds. He would learn how to walk and use his hand again. It might take time, but miracles can happen. Tracey was not going to lose hope and stop fighting. Kost said that he needed to fight, and fight he would.

After the CAT scan, Tracey went directly to Step Down. Fortunately, that afternoon our friend, John, came to visit. I told Tracey that I needed a break and wanted to walk John to the hospital lobby. Shelley stayed with her dad until I returned. When we were a safe distance away, I broke down and told John what had happened. He was incredulous, and agreed that this resident was an asshole. He suggested that I tell Tracey's physicians what had happened. Generally, I am right up front with people and am not afraid of confrontation. However, in Dr. Cauliflower's case, I felt that I needed to keep a safe distance. I was afraid of what I would do, because I knew that ripping his heart out was letting him off too easily.

The next morning, I was able to see Tom Mikkelsen. After I recounted my experience with Dr. Cauliflower, Tom was very apologetic. I told him that I did not expect or need an apology. What I wanted was for Dr. Cauliflower to have a learning experience, so that he would never do the same thing to another patient. I would have talked to him myself, but I was too emotional. I also wanted to make sure that Dr. Cauliflower did not talk to any other family members regarding Tracey. If asked anything, he should refer any questions to Tom or Kost. We then talked about the effects of Tracey's surgery. Yes, there was lack of movement, but only time would tell how much strength Tracey would regain. Tom was not ready to give us a prognosis regarding recovery, for there were still many options that needed to be considered and tried. Yes, this was serious but we were by no means at the end of the road. In the meantime, Tracey would need physical therapy. A social worker would help us make plans.

By the end of Monday, Tracey was moved to a private room. A few close friends came to visit. He tried to smile, but he wore his emotions on his sleeve; he tried to stop himself, but he cried frequently. All I could do was put my arms around him and make sure he knew that he was loved. He wanted to go home and be himself again. The scary part was that he knew that he might never be the same old Tracey again. Normally, he would have been discharged in two days, but he needed physical therapy. He made surprising progress in just three days. However, it wasn't safe for him to come home, and he was too healthy to stay in the hospital.

During rounds, Kost examined Tracey and inspected his face. He didn't understand why there wasn't a noticeable droop. I laughed and said, "You should have known that you couldn't ruin Tracey's good looks." Silently, I thought, "Tracey can recover. If you were wrong about his face, he can recover the use of his left side." I believe that people can overcome seemingly insurmountable obstacles, and I was determined to make Dr. Cauliflower eat his words.

The doctors recommended in-patient physical therapy for three or four weeks. I knew that Tracey would be disappointed that he couldn't come home yet, but he would understand. There were too many obstacles. He needed to be able to walk; he needed to learn how to dress himself using one hand; he needed to build his strength. On Friday, February 10, 1995, he was transferred from Henry Ford Hospital to St. Joseph Mercy Hospital, which was closer to our home.

Chapter Ten

Therapy

We were delayed because the discharge paperwork needed to be completed. It was more complicated than normal, because we needed to take a copy of Tracey's medical history as well as a listing of required medications. By the time we left Henry Ford, it was 1 P.M. Tracey could have been transported by ambulance, but I felt comfortable driving him in our car. It would give us a chance to spend some time alone. Neither one of us had eaten lunch and we had a "Big Mac Attack." We were starving, and it was time for junk food. Since we didn't have a wheelchair, McDonald's drive-thru worked perfectly. We had a picnic in the front seat and enjoyed the sunny day. I didn't think about it at the time, but I don't know what we would have done if Tracey needed to use a rest room.

If we had gone directly to St. Joseph's, we would have arrived in one hour. When we reached admitting, it was almost 3 P.M. Everyone was worried about us. Where had we been? Was something wrong? Apparently, they were expecting us around noon and had been calling Henry Ford and our house trying to find us. We were A.W.O.L. I didn't understand what the fuss was, until I realized that there was a mountain of new paperwork that needed to be completed before the shift change at 4 P.M. Tracey's nurse, Kathy, took it all in stride and helped him get settled.

As we entered the suite where Tracey would stay for the next two weeks, we realized that he would be sharing space with three other patients. They introduced themselves and then allowed us some privacy. However, within thirty minutes everybody was sharing their medical background. It was good therapy for Tracey because he didn't feel quite so sorry for himself. Tom, in the adjacent bed, was experiencing dizziness and had been confined to bed for seven days. They couldn't figure out what was wrong. Everett, a diabetic, was a double leg amputee. George was suffering from weakness due to old age and a bad heart. During the two weeks that they were Tracey's roommates, I never heard any of them complain. They all talked about getting better and going home. Tracey mentioned one day that even though each person was hospitalized for a different reason, they all were very lucky because they had friends and family members who loved and supported them. I was amazed by their positive attitudes. These were remarkable men who set their own fears aside and were genuinely concerned about each other. I also feel that the atmosphere cultivated by the staff at St. Joseph's enabled them to find an inner strength on which to draw.

February is a dreary month in Michigan. The sun rarely shines and it is generally very cold. That year was no exception to the rule. As a result, people are easily depressed. I felt like we were walking on a tightrope. One false move would be disastrous. In addition, I was exhausted and running on empty. I felt like I was treading water with twenty people hanging on to me. I had to make sure that no one drowned. I'm sure that I looked like death warmed over. The dark circles under my eyes looked like a bad make-up artist had gotten hold of me. My days started very early. I continued to work every day until 6 P.M.; then I would go to the hospital and visit until 8 P.M. On the way home, I picked up something to eat, fell into bed, and started all over again the next day. Thank goodness I remained healthy, because I was a prime candidate to catch any virus that was floating around.

Tracey made immediate progress. He needed to be able to climb eight stairs and use the bathroom without assistance. We could see improvement every day. The physical and occupational therapists were like cheerleaders. Every day was filled to the brim and there was very little time for visitors. In the evening, Tracey was exhausted and ready to rest. The days went by quickly, but Tracey couldn't wait until he was able to come home.

I knew that some things in the house needed to be changed in order to make it safe for Tracey. He would need dual railings on our stairway. Otherwise, he would fall. He needed to be able to support himself on the right side when he walked up and down the stairs. A friend, Marty, came to our rescue. Within three days, he designed and installed railings that blended in with the rest of our woodwork. Another friend, Mark, built a ramp so that entry into our house was safe and secure.

After a week of therapy, Tracey received a weekend pass. Luckily, there was not any snow or ice on the ground, because we didn't have an attached garage. Since Tracey was able to walk short distances, we really didn't need a wheelchair. We didn't do much of anything that weekend, and we didn't invite anyone to visit. We just enjoyed some time alone with one another.

Tracey needed to be back at the hospital by 6 P.M. on Sunday. After he was settled in, he was a little depressed. But I reminded him that he would be discharged in four days. Before he knew it, he would be home for good. By the time I returned home, I was exhausted.

There were so many things that needed to be done, as well as appointments to schedule. Tracey's weekend at home had helped us realize to what extent we would need durable medical equipment. His therapists were invaluable, and we depended on their expertise. They are very clever and have a bag of tricks that enable patients to become self-sufficient. By anticipating problems that are not obvious, life is easier for both the patient and their family. There are many types of the same general equipment, but there are various features which can make a big difference. Depending on the patient's challenge, it is mandatory to select the correct supplies. Since Tracey was unable to stand for very long, he needed a chair for the shower. In addition, we wanted to have the flexibility to come and go as we pleased. Even though he could navigate around the house without a problem, we had to have a wheelchair that met important specifications. Last but not least, because his legs had lost strength, a raised toilet seat was essential.

Another area of concern was the furniture in our house. Our sofa would not give Tracey the comfort and support that he needed. I started shopping for a leather lounge chair that would be durable and would complement the couch in our family room. I didn't have any time to waste, so I headed for the local La-Z-Boy store. Within five minutes, I found what I needed. It was probably the fastest purchase that any salesperson almost had. I say almost, because I was informed that we would have to wait three months for delivery. It was not a stock item, and they were not allowed to sell the floor model. They checked the inventory of other stores, but were unable to find the chair I wanted. I was discouraged but not thwarted. My relentless nature came alive. Where there is a will, there is a way. At 9 A.M. the next morning, I called the vice president of manufacturing for La-Z-Boy. I explained my dilemma to his secretary. She was very helpful and sympathetic. Someone would call me back. Two hours later, someone called and listened to my story. He said that he couldn't make any promises, but he would see what he could do. At 1 P.M., the salesperson, who had told me that his general manager had never allowed them to sell a floor model, called me and said, "My manager just gave me the approval. When would you like your chair?" A co-worker volunteered to pick it up in his van after work. By 7 P.M., an azure-blue, leather La-Z-Boy chair was in our family room. A few days later, I personally thanked the general manager for his help. He simply said, "Sometimes exceptions need to be made, especially in family emergencies. We are happy that we could help." This manager had the unselfish courage to make a choice based on human compassion, rather than a business decision based on the bottom line. The stores he managed were in the midst of a huge advertising campaign. The chair he allowed me to purchase was the only one of its type. It was a sacrifice that he was willing to make, because he wanted to help a complete stranger who needed it.

It's amazing how much Tracey improved in such a short period of time. Within four weeks, he went from not being able to move his left side to being able to dress himself partially and walk with a cane. Tracey was determined, but he also had excellent therapists. They challenged him, and he saw that he was making progress. Since it was easy to forget how far he had come, I started to keep a journal. I simply wrote on a calendar all positive changes that occurred. If he was feeling discouraged, I showed him physical proof that he was getting better. This calendar became very important because I also used it to keep track of medications and any other changes that occurred. I was always looking for possible side effects. Once burned, twice wary.

Three days before his discharge, Tracey was very subdued when I visited him. When he and his roommates returned to their room at lunchtime, George's bed had been stripped and he was gone. He had quietly died in his sleep that morning while they had been at therapy. Tracey mentioned that George had said that he didn't think he would be going home. I have read that many people know when they are going to die and many times make a conscious decision when it is time. I did not know George well, but I think he chose to die when his roommates were gone. He knew they were all worried about death, and he wanted to protect them as much as he could.

Everyone kept to themselves that evening. They were all upset. This was the second death Tracey had shared in the past three weeks. It was as if he had been lucky enough to be gone when the Grim Reaper visited. He didn't want to take any chances. He couldn't wait for Thursday to arrive so that he could go home.

As Tracey was counting down the days before he would go home, we needed to schedule the next four weeks of therapy. Just like physicians, occupational and physical therapists have specialties. I found that most are trained in orthopedics, but very few have expertise with brain dysfunction. Since St. Joseph's was forty minutes away, we needed to find a facility that provided the help we needed and at the same time was conveniently located. Transportation was also an issue. Most cab services were not dependable. Luckily, I discovered that St. Joseph's had a satellite office which was ten minutes from our house. Three days a week, family and friends volunteered to pick him up and take him to and from his appointments. Without their help, I would not have been able to work. This also kept Tracey very busy. He was not isolated, and he was able to go out to lunch as well as visit with his friends.

Since I was under a phenomenal amount of stress, I felt like a pressure cooker ready to explode. My optimism for the future was being whittled away. My trust in what others said was minimal. I was almost becoming a convert to the Murphy's Law train of thought: When you think that things can't get worse— watch out! In a way, this skepticism saved us, because insurance coverage was becoming insanely complicated.

I had been religious about checking insurance statements called Explanations of Benefits and making sure that all services were paid. In fact, I discovered over $20,000 in billing and payment errors. I almost had an auditor's mentality. I say almost because I didn't really like what I was doing. I couldn't control the outcome of Tracey's disease, but I was determined that I was not going to undergo a financial nightmare.

Henry Ford Medical Center was "Out of Network." This meant that Tracey's insurance, as the primary insurer, would pay only seventy percent of customary fees for authorized hospitalization, radiation, chemotherapy, and related doctor visits. However, after a $7000 annual deductible was met, one hundred percent was paid. Since Tracey was covered by two insurance policies, we had the luxury of choosing where we wanted treatment. What one company didn't cover, the other would. I thought I understood the intricacies of both policies. I was wrong.

In January 1995, Tracey's employer changed insurance carriers. Coverage basically stayed the same, but Tracey needed to select a new primary care physician. After reviewing a list, we selected Dr. McTurk because his office was convenient. We didn't think much about it until Tracey needed physical, occupational, and speech therapies. I discovered by accident that unless Tracey received a referral from his new primary care physician, therapy would not be covered even though St. Joseph's was considered "In Network."

I was at the end of my rope. I didn't think that Tracey or I could see one more new doctor. I made a few telephone calls and realized that we did not have a choice; we were caught between a rock and a hard place. Fortunately, I talked with Dr. McTurk's administrative assistant, Michelle. I tried to explain our problem. I am amazed she understood one word that I said, because I was sobbing uncontrollably. To say the least, she was wonderful. She took control. We made an appointment to meet with Dr. McTurk so he could give us the referral we needed. We then found out that we would need to see yet another specialist, a physiatrist, in order to extend the prescription for therapy. Over the next nine months, Michelle spent hours providing the documentation that the insurance company required for physical therapy, home care, durable medical equipment, and eventually hospice. On numerous occasions, I thanked Dr. McTurk and Michelle for their help. But like so many others, they simply said, "I wish that there was more that I could do."

As time went on, I became very frustrated dealing with insurance companies. The books explaining benefits did not provide all the facts that I needed. Many times I called and received incorrect information. To make matters worse, I received incomplete details regarding coverage. Sometimes, I would never know what would be paid until I received an Explanation of Benefits. My suggestion to anyone who must deal with insurance companies regarding a major health problem is to request to speak to the same person all the time. Also, get a notebook and log all phone conversations. I did this religiously, and was thankful that I had dates and names along with notes. It came in handy on multiple occasions when problems arose.

With the details of therapy straightened out, Tracey was discharged from St. Joseph's, and we headed back to Henry Ford. When we arrived, we checked our car at valet parking. Tracey was proud of the fact that he was able to walk to our appointment with Dr. Wollner. He had come a long way in a relatively short period of time.

We discussed the recommended chemotherapy plans. Tracey wanted to try the most effective chemo protocol even though it included Procarbazine. He had started to have regrets that he hadn't toughed it out the first time around. Hindsight is a wonderful thing, except it doesn't help or change anything. His physicians were very hesitant about using Procarbazine. They did not want Tracey to have a terrible reaction again. No one really understood why he had become so violently ill. We hoped that the Zofran (nausea medication) would solve the problem. Dr. Wollner brought a new highlight sheet that described potential side effects as well as foods to avoid. I was reading the information, and I suddenly knew why Tracey had been so sick. The brochure said to avoid any foods that contained yogurt. I remembered that Tracey had eaten yogurt to coat his stomach an hour before he took Procarbazine for the first time. I couldn't believe it. No wonder he was so sick. Yogurt was one of the worst possible foods that he could have eaten. He had unknowingly poisoned himself. We kept our fingers crossed as Tracey swallowed the first dose of Procarbazine. Other than being tired, Tracey tolerated the treatment without problems. He would wait two weeks and start the next cycle. His doctors had become very aggressive.

There is an important lesson that anyone who takes prescriptions should learn. Everyone in the medical profession has their specialties. A pharmacist is the best person to talk to regarding drug interactions. Before Tracey took any new medications, I always talked to a hospital pharmacist first. There were not going to be any more problems because we didn't have sufficient or accurate information. Some drugstores now provide data sheets that are very good. However, if you are taking multiple types of drugs, you really need advice based on all your prescriptions. Another important piece of advice is, read instructions carefully. If the label says to take a drug within a certain time frame or to eat/drink with medication, follow the directions exactly. You will probably be able to avoid unnecessary problems. There are always side effects from drugs. Why create extra problems for yourself?

Understandably, Tracey was concerned. He mentioned one day that he felt like he was running out of time and that he needed a miracle. I didn't know what to say. What could I say? Instead, I suggested things that we could do to have fun. It seemed like when things were at their worst, something always happened to lift our spirits. On February 28, a dream of ours came true. I won a trip to Hawaii. For the past year, I had worked very hard to reach my sales quota. I exceeded my goal at the end of February. The reward was an all-expense paid vacation with other sales people who had reached their goals. I was excited because of my personal achievement. In spite of Tracey's illness, I felt like I had lived up to Compuware's trust and had performed at a level that was not only higher than what was expected, but higher than the majority of other sales people. I had not done it on my own. Managers handled sales calls for me when I couldn't attend, and they followed-up on paperwork. But the person who helped me the most was Tracey. I explained to him that he, more than anyone else, was responsible for my success. His encouragement and unselfish courage enabled me to go to work every day. Even though he would have liked me to stay home, he pushed me to travel because he knew that I would not succeed unless I met with my customers face-to-face. After all, he was a salesman. He knew that it took hard work to be successful. He understood my competitive drive. He was proud of me. We had both won this trip and looked forward to going to Hawaii at the end of April.

This good news put new wind in our sails. Tracey started outpatient therapy with new determination. He had two months of hard work and one more cycle of chemo before we headed to our tropical paradise.

The week after his first chemo treatment, Tracey began occupational therapy with Colleen and physical therapy with Lizzy. For the next six months, they rode a roller coaster ride with us from the heights of victory through the valleys of uncertainty. Without their help and encouragement, our lives would have been a disaster. They were as determined as we were, and their efforts made a huge difference. They showed me how I could help at home. Tracey not only needed to gain strength, but he also needed to maintain flexibility. Before exercising, he needed to stretch. Initially, this could take as much as thirty minutes away from therapy, and we couldn't afford to waste precious time. I decided that I would wake up at 5 A.M., get ready for work, and then help Tracey stretch, eat, and dress before his 8 A.M. appointment. It was worth the effort because we could see dramatic improvements. At one point, Tracey was actually able to lope (not quite a gallop) down the hallway. We cried the day that he started to move his fingers. I felt like video taping Tracey's progress and sending it to the doom and gloom resident, Dr. Cauliflower.

Even though he was getting some movement in his hand, his left shoulder was very weak. There was a small separation in his left shoulder, but it was not serious—yet. The weight of his left arm could possibly cause a dislocation. Tracey and I knew from personal experience that we didn't want that to happen. The recommended remedy was more than a sling, it was like a harness. A Velcro cuff, similar to a blood pressure cuff, was wrapped around his left bicep. Three straps were connected and wrapped around the back of his neck, under his right arm and across his chest. I learned that as long as I detached only one strap, I could reconnect this contraption. At first, it was a lot like playing Twister. On a few occasions, I came home to find someone had tried to help Tracey put on the sling. It looked like burglars had tied him up. As usual, he suffered at other peoples' hands with a sense of humor. On a few occasions, Tracey didn't wear the sling, but he paid a price later. His arm became very tired and sore. It became part of our routine to put the sling on first thing in the morning and then take it off at bedtime.

Therapy was very intense and chemotherapy was arduous. Tracey's muscles were as tight as a drum and his energy level was very low. Mentally and physically, we were both exhausted. It was not surprising that it was very difficult for us to relax. It seemed like we were always on guard against a ruthless opponent who used guerrilla warfare tactics. We had to be constantly vigilant—ready and armed before the next attack. In trying to find ways to relieve our tension, we discovered a secret weapon: body massage. Every two weeks, Randy, a professional masseur, came to our home and worked miracles. Frequently, we fell asleep while soft music played in the background. I was always amazed that Randy was able to help us relax physically and emotionally—no matter how agitated or tense we were. As I came to realize the importance and power of the human touch, this luxury quickly became a necessity. Massage renewed our spirits and raised our energy levels so that we could face a silent enemy. Eventually, its healing powers became critical in our lives and saved us when we didn't know where else to turn.

Toward the end of March, Tracey became fairly independent through hard work. He was determined to be in shape for our Hawaii trip. Since it was safe for him to be home alone during the day, I was able to go to work. However, we did have one obstacle to overcome. I needed to travel for some major client presentations and Tracey could not be alone at night. Our next door neighbors, Ron and Linda, Tracey's Aunt Dorothy, and our friend, Jan, came to our rescue. They volunteered to spend the night. This was not an easy task, because they also had to help Tracey shower, dress, fix his meals, and transport him to therapy. Without their help, I would have had to quit my job. When I had to leave town on business, I was very nervous. Everything worked out, but the first morning there was a problem. Linda had to cook. She was not known for her culinary skill, but I thought oatmeal would be within her abilities. I put out everything she would need, including what I thought were easy to follow directions—"Just add water and cook in the microwave for 2 minutes." Linda was fine until she realized that she had to measure the ingredients. The oatmeal was not in a packet. She was worried and with good reason. When she pulled the bowl out of the microwave, she had a miniature bowling ball. Ron gave it a shot without any better success. They all had a great laugh and then rummaged through the cupboard for some Cheerios.

Another day, Tracey and Aunt Dorothy decided to go to the movies. As long as he used a cane, Tracey could walk independently. They bought popcorn and a soda to share. Aunt Dorothy headed off toward the theater. Suddenly, she heard a voice calling her name saying, "What about me?" She turned around and was more than a little embarrassed. She had walked off carrying Tracey's cane and left him holding their snack. Humorous incidents like these became part of Tracey's repertoire. I heard them repeated many times, each time a little different than the last. Tracey enjoyed entertaining people with his adventures and was famous for making them bigger and better. He embellished so much that friends often scratched their heads and wondered, "Was I really there when that happened?"

By the beginning of April, our days settled into a fairly normal routine. I noticed that Tracey was having problems with his short term memory. At first, I thought it was because he didn't have a regular schedule, or it was yet another side effect of the medication. I realized that every day I had to remind him a couple of times what we were going to do, but even then he might not remember. I mentioned this to Colleen and Lizzy. Apparently, this is a common problem with any patient who has suffered brain trauma of any kind. In Tracey's case, it was surgery. The brain is a marvelous organ. Through repetition and hard work, people can relearn how to think and put ideas together. Tracey's physiatrist, Dr. Sesi, recommended speech therapy in order to help Tracey improve his memory and made a referral through Dr. McTurk. I had learned my lesson and would follow the insurance rules. And so now Tracey began work with Ruth, a speech therapist.

During the second week of April, we were riding the crest of the wave when it started to crash. Out of nowhere, Tracey started having problems with his balance. One day, he was sitting in a chair without arm rests. He began to lean to the side, couldn't catch himself, and fell on the floor. Luckily, there were only bruises. Suddenly, he was very unsteady on his feet. As a result, he became frightened of the stairs. He had been doing so well. What was the matter? There were so many potential causes. In ten days, we were supposed to leave for Hawaii. I didn't know if Tracey would overcome the disappointment if we couldn't go. I called Tom Mikkelsen, and he wanted to test the Dilantin level in Tracey's blood. The results showed that the daily dosage needed to be lowered. It would take five days for the level to adjust. We kept our fingers crossed. As each day passed, Tracey's balance improved. Even though he couldn't walk without someone's assistance, he was much better.

Lizzy noticed muscle deterioration during physical therapy, so she arranged to have a leg brace made for Tracey. He was having a hard time lifting his left toes when he walked. As a result, he was tripping. The brace gave his ankle and foot additional support so that he could walk with less effort. We saw an immediate improvement, but Tracey would not use the brace when he wore shorts. I didn't want to fight with him. I understood that it brought back childhood memories of his battle to recover from polio. He didn't want to think of himself as an invalid and couldn't stand the stares from inconsiderate people. I enlisted the help of Colleen and Lizzy. Maybe they could convince Tracey to wear the brace. They were a little confused, because Tracey had not resisted wearing the arm brace which supported his left shoulder. Their comment was, "We don't understand why Tracey is rebelling. What's the difference?" I explained that Tracey was afraid of being considered a cripple. He perceived the arm support as a sling. After all, that's what they called it. But the leg brace was called a leg brace. They talked with Tracey, and explained that he needed the brace not only for support but for safety reasons. He was catching his toe with every step. It was only a matter of time before he fell. He could be seriously injured. It was a temporary measure, and once he gained some muscle strength in his leg, he wouldn't need the brace anymore. When I came home that evening, Tracey was wearing shorts and his leg brace. He never complained again.

Initially, I was given a ten second demonstration on how to slide Tracey's foot into his tennis shoe while he was wearing the brace. It was pretty tricky, because it was very snug and there was a hinge on the back of the ankle. It had a mind of its own, and the hinge was worse than any pit bull. Its jaws would snap and attack its unsuspecting victims whose only sin was that they were trying to help Tracey get dressed. Any attempt to struggle would incite the vicious beast to bear down harder. It was in control, and would release when it was good and ready. Due to my lightning fast reflexes, I had escaped injury. One day, I must have been in a fog because it trapped me. Tracey was helpless. Every time he moved, I screamed louder. Finally, it took pity on me and its vice grip unlocked. The brace was strapped onto Tracey's leg. Otherwise, it would have been out the window. However, as it left my hand, his shoe ricocheted out of the bedroom and down the stairway like a speeding bullet. Had I been able to control its direction, any baseball manager would have recruited me as a fastball pitcher. I was a lunatic and Tracey helplessly watched me. He had a forlorn look on his face, but he didn't say anything. I took a deep breath and looked at my injury. It hurt worse than it looked. The skin on my hand had been pinched. It was red, but there was no blood. To say the least, I was a little embarrassed by my temper tantrum. Tracey had the good sense not to say anything until I returned with his shoe. He commented, "Maybe I won't wear the brace today." However, I was not going to be defeated by a piece of plastic. I would just be more careful. Eventually, I learned that the safest time to put Tracey's shoe on was while he laid flat on the bed. This way, the hinge was less likely to bite me.

Our departure date for Hawaii was Thursday, April 27. On Monday, April 24, we knew that we were going. The day before we left, Tracey had a CAT scan, but we decided that we did not want to know the results until after we returned from our vacation. Nothing was going to spoil our dream come true.

Chapter Eleven

Dreams Do Come True

With bags packed and tickets in hand, we boarded the airplane. Destination: Kauai, Hawaii. Beforehand, I had talked to D'Arcie in Compuware's travel department about our special needs. She made arrangements for bulkhead seats, a wheelchair, a hotel room that was centrally located, and a shower chair. She made sure that we had everything we needed to have a wonderful vacation.

Most of the people that I worked with knew that Tracey had been battling brain cancer. They had not seen him since December, and I know they were shocked by how weak he had become in such a short time. Everyone was aware that occasionally we needed help, and they were more than willing to do anything. All we had to do was ask. However, the one thing we didn't want was anyone feeling sorry for us. Pity was not our cup of tea. We were there to enjoy ourselves like everyone else. Our positive attitude enabled us to become just part of the group and have a good time.

Our flight was very long but fairly uneventful. The only major obstacle was using the bathroom. Tracey was not stable enough to walk alone, with or without a cane. Once we were in the aisle, I walked backward and he grasped both my forearms. We slowly inched our way to our destination, which was about six feet away. As we approached the door, we turned counterclockwise so that Tracey could back into the lavatory. I followed and the flight attendant closed the door behind us. We were wedged in a two by four closet. If the door opened unexpectedly, I would have popped out like a jack-in-the-box. Tracey was sitting and I had a leg up on the sink. We both started to laugh. Where was our camera when we needed it? As we exited, we noticed some shocked faces and a few people whispering. We laughed even harder. They thought that we were members of the "Mile High Club," and the flight attendants were helping us with our little rendezvous.

On arrival, we received the traditional Hawaiian lei and headed to our hotel. There was a reception that evening. We excused ourselves early and headed to bed. It had been a long day. Since breakfast for the group was scheduled for 7:30 A.M., every day began at 5 A.M. for me and 6 A.M. for Tracey. We needed to continue with his stretching exercises. Even though his balance was better, he could not walk anywhere without help. This meant that at least twice during the night, I got up with Tracey to help him go to the bathroom. Neither one of us was getting an uninterrupted night's sleep, and it was becoming a problem. We tried limiting fluids at night but it made no difference. Maybe it was the drugs. We'd check with the doctors when we returned to Michigan.

There were many planned and optional activities for the group. I was concerned that Tracey would be depressed because he couldn't play golf. The weather was perfect, and he loved the adventure of conquering a new course. This one was a TPC course—a private course designed for tournament play for the worlds top professional golfers. We talked about it, but he was more concerned that he was holding me back and spoiling my fun. I agreed that golf would have been fun, but only if we could have played together. We were there to have fun with each other, and playing a round of golf wasn't that important to me. I didn't want to do anything that we couldn't share.

The next six days were filled with sightseeing, lounging, dancing, and fun. One of the highlights of the trip was taking a tour by helicopter. The view was spectacular, and the guide gave a fascinating commentary on the history and geography of the island. Tracey sat in the cockpit next to the pilot. As he was leaning over to take a photo of the breathtaking scenery, we hit an air pocket. The adjective "disposable" had new meaning as our camera dropped a thousand feet into the canyon below. Oh well, our memories were far more spectacular than any pictures would be, and what a story this would be for Tracey to tell! In any event, I had a reputation as an amateur photographer, because I had disposable cameras (flash, telephoto, underwater, and wide angle) for every occasion. My purse weighed fifty pounds, but we would have lots of pictures despite the loss of one camera. Not only were our photos beautiful, but they also captured our happiness. No matter where we were or what we were doing, we were smiling.

One of the questions that people asked us was, "What do you remember the most about Hawaii?" We talked about the helicopter ride, but personally I thought about something more memorable. One evening, we went to a luau. The men wore tropical shirts and the women wore wraparound muumuus. Tracey decided that he wanted to dance. By the time we reached the dance floor, the band was playing fast music. We decided to sit down and rest for a minute. While we were watching the crowd, we heard a scream and saw a flash of fabric falling. A woman, who shall remain anonymous, had lost her muumuu. I guess she hadn't used a safety pin in a strategic place. Eventually, the music changed. I don't remember the melody they played, but I do remember that it was last time Tracey held me in his arms to slow dance.

Our last evening in Kauai, we attended a formal dinner. It was a black tie affair. All of the sales people were honored for their achievements. When my name was announced, I accepted an award that was as much Tracey's as it was mine. There was more dancing that evening, but Tracey and I were too tired. The busy week was finally catching up to us. Besides, tomorrow was going to be a long day. By the time we went to bed, we fell asleep as soon as our heads hit our pillows.

The red-eye flight back to Michigan was grueling. We walked into our house at 9 A.M. on Thursday, May 4. Reality would meet us all too soon. We had an appointment with Dr. Wollner the next afternoon. Our reprieve was over. Chemo was scheduled to begin again the following week.

Chapter Twelve

Coming Back to Reality

Thursday, Tracey slept most of the day. It seemed like the flight home from Hawaii took everything out of him. The twenty-two hour ordeal made him so physically exhausted that he had no desire to eat. In the afternoon, I noticed that his left leg and ankle were swollen. He had been sitting for a long time, and I thought that his leg brace had cut off his circulation. I massaged his leg every couple of hours and raised it with a pillow. By Friday morning, the swelling disappeared. Since Tracey's appointment with Dr. Wollner was at 1:30 P.M., I went to work. At noon, Tracey's dad dropped him off at my office, and we headed to Henry Ford Hospital.

We were becoming familiar faces to the staff at Henry Ford. Since Tracey was no longer able to walk very far, we always used valet parking. Some people may think valet service is a luxury, but for us it was a necessity. We needed easy access and protection from bad weather. Hospital wheelchairs were readily available so that I didn't need to retrieve ours from the truck. Even though we had a lightweight model, our wheelchair was still heavy and awkward to lift. Recently, we had begun to be greeted by staff, who offered assistance and whisked Tracey off to wherever he needed to go for his appointment. This service made a huge difference for both Tracey and me. Transfers in and out of the car were easier and safer. In addition, it took some of the burden off my shoulders. I was beginning to feel physically overwhelmed, and any helping hand was appreciated. Some people might have suggested that I ask family or friends to help. However, Tracey and I needed to face his doctors alone. We couldn't deal with other people's fears. We had only enough strength for each other. Although we were now familiar with where the various departments were located, I'm sure that navigating around the hospital was confusing for most patients, to say the least. Visiting doctors in a hospital is very stressful, especially when you are always bracing yourself against bad news. Unexpected kindness from strangers is a potent prescription to help alleviate this natural anxiety.

It was easy to remember where we needed to go, because the Oncology Clinic was located on the thirteenth (yes, that's right) floor. We tried to schedule most of our appointments for immediately after lunch. This eliminated the tedious waiting that sometimes occurred. Everyone who had an appointment was fighting for his or her life, and occasionally patients needed to be seen immediately. This meant that sometimes there were double and triple bookings. If you had to wait an hour, you tried to wait patiently. After all, there might be an instance when you needed extra time with your doctor. There was an unspoken code among patients and their families—no one should be rushed just to adhere to the doctor's appointment schedule.

It always surprised me that we were recognized by the staff, because this department was very busy. At first, I thought we were familiar faces because we had been seeing Dr. Wollner approximately every six weeks for eighteen months. However, I came to realize that these compassionate individuals made an effort to know us. They understood that their patients needed to be recognized as human beings who wanted to survive, and who had dreams that they wanted to come true. Tracey was more than just a medical record number. On this particular day, the receptionist asked Tracey how he was feeling. She did not ignore the fact that his condition had changed, and made mention that she noticed he had been doing better a few months ago. We were not offended by her candor because she was genuinely concerned. We appreciated the fact that she perceived that things were different. On the other hand, we both had recently noticed that some friends and acquaintances did not know what to say and did not want to hear that everything was not okay. It made them feel uncomfortable. In response, I had stopped talking about Tracey's failing health. I could tell by their faces that they didn't want to hear. I simply started saying, "He's hanging in there," and I would change the subject. I didn't have the energy to make everyone else feel better.

As Dr. Wollner entered the examining room, I know that we were both holding our breath. He was pleased that Tracey had tolerated the first two chemo sessions. We mentioned the frequent urination problem. Tracey was now waking up at least four times every night and needed to urinate every couple of hours during the day. The cause was probably a side effect of the steroids. We explained that a urinal at night was not a solution because I would still need to get up and help Tracey. Besides, there was always backwash. Any man who has tried to use a urinal in bed knows that backwash means you need to change all of your bed linen. Fortunately, Dr. Wollner suggested the use of a condom catheter. We had talked to at least five other people, and we had never heard about this device. We had been persistent enough to continue to ask for help until someone came up with an idea that might provide a solution. Neither one of us was getting any sleep. We'd get a prescription and give it a shot, because we were willing to try anything. With that problem addressed, we asked about the results of the CAT scan taken eight days prior. Dr. Wollner left the room for a couple of minutes. When he returned, he quietly told us that the preliminary report indicated that there was recurrence. He didn't know all the details. In the blink of an eye, our dream turned into a nightmare. Chemo would be postponed until after we met with our neurosurgeon. We already had a follow-up appointment for the following Thursday with Kost. We were in shock. Tracey's last surgery was only three months ago. How could the tumor have come back so soon? We left in a trance. Neither one of us said much during the hour drive home.

As soon as we walked in the door, I called our lifeline—Tom Mikkelsen—who had ordered the scan. What did he know? I couldn't believe my luck when I caught him at his desk at 5 P.M. on a Friday afternoon. No, he hadn't seen the results yet. He mentioned that recently he had two brain tumor patients whose scans appeared to show tumor recurrence. However, it turned out that the patients only had scarring and swelling from the surgery. His advice was, "Don't jump to any conclusions." They would have the final results next week. We would discuss them at our Thursday appointment with Kost.

We tried to have a positive outlook, but we were both angry and irritable. Reality had slapped us across the face. Once again, we were in the wait and see mode.

On Monday, Tracey went to therapy bearing Hawaiian gifts—chocolate-covered macadamia nuts. Within thirty seconds, Colleen knew that something was wrong. We spent the next hour telling Colleen, Lizzy, and Ruth the disappointing news. We were trying to be hopeful, but we were on an emotional roller-coaster that wouldn't stop to let us off. Just being able to talk was a relief.

We were now faced with a new dilemma. I needed to continue to work, but Tracey could no longer stay home alone. For Tracey's safety and my peace of mind, we couldn't totally rely on our family and friends. We needed professional help and had to enter into the complicated world of home care. Having already learned our lesson about insurance rules and regulations, I called Michelle at Dr. McTurk's office. Within a few hours, a nurse scheduled an interview for Tuesday morning so that we would have assistance in our home by Friday.

In an effort to stay organized, I had a summary of Tracey's medical history. It included the names, phone numbers, and specialties of all his physicians, his diagnosis, treatments, prescriptions, insurance information, emergency phone numbers, and most important—an advance directive, or "Designation of Patient Advocate Form."

In Michigan, in order to ensure that your wishes regarding medical treatment are followed, anyone eighteen years of age or older should complete a document called a "Designation of Patient Advocate Form," commonly referred to as an advance directive. It becomes legally effective if you are unable to participate in medical treatment decisions. You may list specific care and treatment you do or do not want, and you appoint someone to act for you regarding your care, custody, and treatment. This document is free, completely separate from a will or durable power of attorney, does not require the assistance of a lawyer, and can be changed or modified at any time. All hospitals and physicians have these forms available. It simplifies the decision-making process for both your family and your physicians. This way you have express, conclusive evidence of your healthcare wishes.

Since I had all this information readily available, we could concentrate on our specific home care needs. A word of warning: home care organizations do not explain, and are not responsible for explaining, insurance benefits. It was my understanding that our coverage included one hundred days of support, and that there was a minimum billable time of four hours. As long as Tracey continued with therapy three times a week, we would only need an aide for five hours on Mondays, Wednesdays, and Fridays. On Tuesdays and Thursdays, we would need someone from 7:30 A.M. until 6:30 P.M., or eleven hours. Initially, I didn't understand that the insurance company interpreted one day as only four hours. If we needed an aide for five hours, that was considered two full days, or eight hours. On the one hand, we were forced to use two days of Tracey's benefit, but on the other hand, the home care agency was paid for only five hours. At this rate, Tracey's home care benefit would expire in eight weeks instead of twenty weeks. This is "managed healthcare." It is the method insurance companies use to reduce or manage healthcare costs. At thirteen dollars an hour, home care was going to cost us at least $500 per week by the middle of June.

My head began to throb. Healthcare costs were skyrocketing. Insurance premiums, prescriptions, and home care costs would exceed $2,300 per month. To make matters worse, I didn't see how I was going to be able to continue in my sales position. I didn't see how I would be able to travel. I felt like the child in the poem about the leak in the dike. I had my finger jammed in the hole, but the wall was beginning to split like a spider web. I was going to be washed away in a flood of debt. To make matters worse, Shelley's college tuition was due.

Life had handed us a deck of cards that was too big to manage. I had two alternatives. Leave the game or split the deck. Even though I would have liked to run away and have all my problems disappear, leaving was not a choice. I decided to take one card at a time. The first card was our meeting with Kost on Thursday. Hopefully, we wouldn't draw a joker.

Chapter Thirteen

Jokers are Wild

We were nervous wrecks by the time the alarm went off at 3 A.M. on Thursday morning. In order to be on time for our 8 A.M. appointment, we needed to leave by 6:45 A.M. I had to shower and dress for work as well as get Tracey ready. There was no time for breakfast. I would not even let Tracey have a cup of coffee. He was still having bladder problems, and we had at least an hour-long drive in rush hour traffic. I was on edge; Tracey was cranky. We were a disaster waiting to happen. Generally, Tracey was pretty talkative in the morning. Today, neither one of us was saying too much. We were trying to save our inner resources for our meeting with Kost.

We left the house right on time. As with all good plans, the unavoidable happened. Tracey had to go to the bathroom. Luckily, we stopped at a gas station that did not have any obstacles and had handicapped facilities. Even so, this unscheduled stop took twenty minutes. We were running late. I hated being late. I was losing control of everything. Our life was falling apart and there was nothing that I could do. I know that I was being unreasonable. So what if we were late? It was not the end of the world. After all, how many times had we waited for a doctor? They could wait for us one time. My normal common sense was evaporating, and there was nothing I could do. Tracey watched and waited. He was not saying anything. Something had to give soon or we both were going to explode. It was then that we were dealt a joker.

We pulled up to valet parking and still had twenty minutes before our appointment. My cousin Jake was waiting for us. He had come to work early so that he could help. I hopped out of the truck and asked for a wheelchair. In order to prevent theft, hospital wheelchairs were chained together and locked every evening. Unfortunately for us, no one knew where the key was. I was furious. Jake left in search of a wheelchair, but I was impatient. I was not going to be late. I was wearing high heels and a pale yellow suit, and as I struggled to pull the wheelchair out of the back of our truck, the wheelchair brushed against my clothes. I could have been mistaken for a bumble bee because my suit was now black and yellow. My temper was at a boiling point. I think I probably would have been admitted to the hospital at that moment if someone had taken my blood pressure. I transferred Tracey from the truck to the wheelchair. I had the good sense to put on the wheelchair's brakes, but I forgot that Tracey could not feel that his left arm was dangling to the side. However, he was able to feel his hand being pinched as I attempted to swing the foot rest in place. Needless to say, he screamed at me, "Would you stop being in such a goddamn hurry!" I moved his arm out of harm's way, but the foot rest would not stay in place. I attempted to hold it in place with my foot. Instead, I bent it into the asphalt. The wheelchair was not going anywhere anytime soon. I was my own worst enemy. I was unable to think anymore. I could only react. My right leg came back, and my aim was accurate. As my high-heeled shoe met the wheelchair, metal flew. Now we were totally disabled. A traffic jam was developing in valet parking. There must have been five cars waiting, and then, someone honked their horn. My arms dropped to my side and I began to sob. I am sure everyone was wondering if I was the patient. Just then Jake rushed up, got down on his hands and knees in his suit and fixed the wheelchair so that it would move. I was beyond caring what anyone thought. Jake patted me on the back and said, "Come on. Let's go." By the time we reached the eleventh floor, I had calmed down. Remarkably, we were right on time. It was 8 A.M. We were directed to a room to wait. Kost had never been late. Today, we waited thirty minutes.

Jake was trying to break the icy silence. He started an idle conversation. He would take the wheelchair to a welder in the hospital and try to have it fixed during our appointment. Tracey and I were just starting to relax when Kost arrived. Jake excused himself and left with the wheelchair. Kost was perplexed. He didn't say anything but I know he was thinking, "Why is he leaving with Tracey's wheelchair?" Now it was Tracey's turn to get even. With a twinkle in his eyes, he proudly announced, "She's abusing me Kost. Kathy kicked and broke the wheelchair in the parking lot. And I was in it!" I must have turned fifty shades of red. They both were staring at me. There was nowhere to go, nowhere to hide. It was my turn to defend myself. What could I say? Should I claim temporary insanity? Instead, I shrugged my shoulders and said, "What can I say? So far, it hasn't been a very good day!" We all laughed. Now we could focus on the reason we were meeting. There was definitely a thaw, but we were still walking on thin ice.

I recited a litany of all the things that had been going wrong. Tracey was weaker and his balance was terrible. He could not monitor the volume of his voice. His short term memory was awful. We were not getting any sleep because he was going to the bathroom every two hours. The scariest change was that Tracey had lost some peripheral vision in his right eye. Kost checked Tracey's reflexes, strength and vision. Then, I remembered the primary reason for our visit. "What are the CAT scan results? When we talked to Dr. Wollner, he told us that there is recurrent tumor." It was immediately evident that there was a communication problem. Kost seemed surprised, and did not know that Tracey had even had a scan. I had assumed incorrectly that he had been told. I never assumed anything again. It might have been irritating, but from then on I called each physician when I felt there was a change or a test result that they needed to review.

Kost excused himself and left for ten minutes. When he returned, his eyes looked very tired and his shoulders were slightly stooped. He sat toe-to-toe with Tracey. He had read the report, but had not seen the scan itself. The facts were, "There is a tumor in the left front brain. Surgery is not an option, but a one time high dosage of radiation, called radiosurgery, is possible. This new course of treatment needs to be approved by the tumor board. Hopefully, the procedure can be scheduled for next week." He waited for us to absorb this new information. For the first time since the original prognosis, I was mute. I felt as if I had fallen through the ice. I was drowning. All I could do was blink my eyes. Did Tracey comprehend what Kost had just said? Tracey began asking questions. He understood all too well. Not only was the tumor back, but it had spread from the right side of the brain to the left. The new tumor was affecting his vision. He had already lost the use of his left side. What else was he going to lose? Fortunately, Kost felt the risk was minimal. Did we have any more questions? Tracey shook his head no and said, "Let's do this as soon as possible."

Tracey had complete trust in whatever Kost recommended. I could not say a word. Kost stood and opened the door to leave. I held my head in my hand and began to sob. The door shut. Kost sat down and put his hand on mine. Even though his touch was unexpected, this time I did not pull away. The defenses that protected my comfort zone had disappeared. I was unable to think. I felt like an empty shell. For a couple of minutes, no one said anything. Then Kost patted my hand and said, "You know Kathy, you have to stop kicking wheelchairs in the parking lot." I started to laugh through my tears. I shook my head, "It's not fair. Tracey is behaving himself. For the first time in our marriage, he is doing everything that I tell him to do. Only it hasn't made any difference." The tension was broken. It made no sense, but we were laughing through our pain so that we could move on and make decisions. Kost excused himself and said that he would be back in a minute. When he returned, he brought reinforcements. Tom Mikkelsen joined us.

Kost and Tom stood in the doorway while Tracey and I sat on either side. Kost looked exhausted and had passed the baton to Tom. They were trying to share their strength and provide encouragement. Tom took a philosophical approach. He began by saying, "In the course of treatment, you constantly need to watch for changes and adjust your strategy. The path you choose can change many times, and after awhile it ages you." He had my attention. I was no longer mute. In fact, I swatted his arm with the back of my right hand. I had startled him. I guess it's not every day that the wife of a patient hits the doctor. I chuckled and pretended to be offended. "You know Tom, you sure know how to build a woman's ego. Are you telling me that I look older since you met me a year ago?" He was taken off guard and started to apologize. I was laughing. "Tom, I was only kidding." Humor had returned. I was okay. We talked for a few more minutes. We needed to talk again after the tumor board approved the recommendation. I would call tomorrow. As we were preparing to leave, Jake arrived with Tracey's wheelchair. Thankfully, it had been repaired, and we headed home—totally exhausted.

Friday morning arrived and so did Russ, the first home care aide. I had planned to work from home because I did not want to leave Tracey alone with a stranger. You hear horror stories about the healthcare industry, and I did not want to take any chances. Russ and I talked for about thirty minutes. He seemed pleasant enough, but I felt uneasy for some reason. I could not put my finger on it. It was time for Tracey to start his day. I thought it would be a good idea to show Russ what our daily routine was like. I was not thinking very clearly. I was not putting myself in Tracey's shoes. Instead of letting them get to know one another over breakfast, their introduction started with a shower and stretching exercises. Tracey did not complain, but he later told me that he was very uncomfortable. A complete stranger was helping him with personal hygiene and physical therapy before they had a chance to say, "Hello." Generally, I felt that I was a very sensitive person, but I had been so involved in finding a solution that I had inadvertently caused a problem. Other than being concerned with his personal safety, we needed an aide to help Tracey exercise. Russ apparently had some experience working with stroke patients who had similar physical limitations. I demonstrated stretching movements with Tracey's hand, arm, foot, and leg. Russ seemed eager to help. He repeated the same routines, but then he started to vary them and add some of his own without asking. Now I was concerned. Tracey's therapists had taken time to show me effective ways to help Tracey build his strength. They had stressed that there were certain exercises that could be detrimental. I wanted someone who had initiative, but not someone who would make therapy decisions. Russ was only scheduled for the morning. When he left, Tracey looked at me and said, "What do you think?" I wanted Tracey to make decisions so I deferred to him. "It's more important to know what you think. Russ seems okay. But, if you don't like him, we will find someone else." Tracey looked relieved and sighed, "I don't like him. He makes me feel uncomfortable. Besides, he has dirty finger nails." I was disappointed that the first aide did not work out. When I called the agency, they were understanding and agreed to schedule someone else.

I called Tom Mikkelsen on Friday afternoon to finalize details for the radiosurgery. Apparently, he was embarrassed by what he had said the previous day. He began our conversation by apologizing. I interrupted, "I was only kidding, Tom. It was a joke." We moved on to more pressing issues. The tumor board had approved the radiation treatment. In order to complete and coordinate all the necessary plans, we would need to wait two weeks. Tracey needed a new test called a brain SPECT (single photon emission computed tomography). It would give them additional information for tracking the tumor. It was scheduled for Monday morning. Wednesday afternoon we would meet with Dr. Kim, the radiation oncologist, and then with Kost, the neurosurgeon. At the end of our conversation, we reviewed the plan and I started to philosophize about the treatment of brain tumors. "You know, Tom, I've learned over the past year that change is inevitable. First, you take one path and then another until it . . . " Tom interrupted me this time, "I'm never going to live this down am I?" "Probably not, Tom. But have a nice weekend."

We tried to maintain as normal a schedule as possible. Tracey continued going to therapy even though he was gradually losing strength. The home care agency assigned a young woman named Peggy. She seemed very industrious. A full-time college student, she planned to attend law school. Her experience included working with severely disabled patients, who for the most part, were confined to bed and could not talk. I quickly realized that working for us was like a vacation compared to other assignments. Fortunately, Tracey liked Peggy and felt safe with her. If Tracey started to lose his balance, she could grasp and stabilize him with one arm. She was very strong, but she was also very pregnant—six months pregnant. I was concerned, but her doctor had approved her ability to work until the middle of July. I decided that I could only worry short term. We would resolve home care issues as they arose. In the meantime, we had the good fortune to have Peggy working for us.

As each day passed, Tracey and I became more nervous. Radiosurgery was a relatively new procedure and sounded simple. However, there were many variables. There was no room for any mechanical or human errors. Otherwise, Tracey's life was in jeopardy. Once again, we had to trust his physicians and their expertise. We knew that preparation was very complex and sophisticated. Over the weekend we decided to help, and designed a piece of equipment to simplify the process. On the left side of a helmet, we painted a bullseye with four strategically placed arrows which gave directions to "RADIATE HERE!" By the time we finished our creation, we were laughing hysterically. Tracey couldn't wait to show off his protective head gear. Over the past year, he felt that he had gained medical knowledge and expertise from his personal experience on the surgeon's table. Why not share his high-tech discovery? But before our appointments on Wednesday, Tracey had cold feet. He wasn't sure that his doctors would share our sense of humor. It was one thing to joke with each other, but he didn't want to offend the specialists who were treating him. Tracey did not want to take any chances. The helmet stayed in the car. As it turned out, it would not have been a problem, because we talked about our innovative invention and everyone laughed.

Although we had been able to keep our sense of humor, we both knew that the appearance of a new tumor site meant that this insidious disease was gaining control. We were both worried. Each night before we went to sleep, Tracey and I had the habit of talking about our day. We treasured this quiet time together because there were no distractions. After I had turned out the lights and crawled into bed, we held hands for a moment and then Tracey whispered, "Have you ever thought about me dying?" Neither one of us had been able to talk about death in the light of day. Perhaps, in a way, darkness made us feel safe and protected us from the fear that we would see in each other's eyes. My body was rigid, and then my emotions exploded in a rush of tears. I tried to comfort both of us by wrapping my arms around Tracey. I laid my head on his chest and sobbed, "Yes, I've thought about it. You're my best friend. I don't know what I'd do without you. I don't want to lose you." I couldn't see his reaction, but I could feel his body relax. He sighed, "I feel like I need a miracle. My time is running out." Tracey needed something from me. I couldn't cure his cancer, but I could reassure him. "Tracey, I love you. You are my heart and soul. We will fight this thing together. I will always be with you—no matter what happens." We held on to one another. Finally, sleep offered us a temporary escape.

Before we knew it, the day for the radiosurgery arrived. Since most of the day would be spent waiting for the operation to occur, I told our families and friends that I would call them with updates during the day. Neither Tracey nor I had the energy to comfort or visit with anyone. Everyone respected our wishes and allowed us the leeway we needed. We arrived at Henry Ford Hospital at 6 A.M. on Thursday, May 27. Forty-five minutes later, Kost was searching for Tracey. There was no time to waste, because a number of procedures needed to be completed if surgery was going to occur that evening. The schedule was very tight. I was told to wait. About twenty minutes later, Kost was searching for me. He wanted to give me Tracey's eyeglasses. This gave me an opportunity to talk with him privately. I hadn't really asked any direct questions about the results of the last CAT scan.

I took a deep breath and confirmed, "You are only radiating the new tumor site. Is it true that the tumor has also reappeared in the original site?" Kost nodded his head. I couldn't talk any more. My eyes were brimming and tears slowly dropped. I must have looked forlorn because as he turned to leave, Kost said, "Kathy, I'm not going to desert Tracey." I nodded and sighed, "Yes, Kost, I know, and so does Tracey." I was reminded once again that we were not fighting this war on our own.

Suddenly Ann Lucente, Kost's nurse associate, appeared. She had forgotten all about me. I wasn't sure what to expect when I saw Tracey. At first glance, he looked like he belonged on Star Trek, for his head gear looked like something from another galaxy. He had been drugged so he was definitely a little spacey. I'm not sure he appreciated my humor, but I told him, "You look like Darth Vader wearing night vision goggles." Later, he described what had transpired. First, a halo literally needed to be screwed into his head. If you can imagine positioning a human skull in the center ring of a Christmas tree stand with four screws, you will be able to picture this device in your mind's eye. He couldn't feel anything as Kost turned the screws, but Tracey said, "The local anesthesia hurt like hell! Ann told me to hold her hand. I squeezed so hard I thought that I would break her hand."

The next step was to undergo another CAT scan. As we waited for the x-ray equipment to become available, I was able to see the tender care Tracey was receiving, especially from Ann. A few minutes ago, she had shared her strength when he needed it. Now her gentle touch and good humor had a soothing effect. We were both able to relax. We could trust these people, because they possessed the unselfish courage to care about him as a person.

When Tracey had been positioned for the CAT scan, Kost was paged so that he could check the alignment. The halo which encircled Tracey's forehead was used as a point of reference. In this way, they could direct the radiation to the correct location in the brain. After reviewing the results of the CAT scan and the physicians' treatment plan, a physicist made the necessary adjustments to the radiation equipment. Then the computer was programmed to radiate the tumor site. A millimeter error was unacceptable. Perfection was essential. I know that every procedure which Tracey had successfully survived was very complicated. However, this surgery was invisible to the naked eye. In the end, his physicians needed to rely on the data provided by computers in order to make a decision to proceed. What if there was a technical failure? Now, we not only had to trust a team of people, but we also had to trust the information provided by a machine. Technology is amazing, but it's scary at the same time.

By noon, there was nothing we could do but wait. Even though Tracey did not relish the idea, he decided that he needed a catheter. Since he had received a tranquilizer, he felt that it would be safer if he didn't need to walk to the bathroom. In addition, once he was positioned for the radiosurgery, he would not be able to move.

At 4 P.M., Tracey was transported by ambulance to a satellite clinic where the radiation equipment was located. There were at least ten specialists involved—technicians, nurses, doctors, and physicists. Each person had a critical role in ensuring the success of this delicate operation. We arrived at 5:30 P.M.; Tracey was positioned on a hard metal table, and his head was locked into place. An hour passed. During this time, my friend Kay appeared. She suggested playing cards, but I declined. She understood that I needed to be calm and quiet. We talked a little, but mostly I sat and tapped my foot. Before the actual surgery, the computer executed multiple practice runs. I was told that it generally did not take this long, but the computer data indicated that some adjustments were needed. Until the correct modifications had been made and everyone was satisfied, they did not want to proceed. I was in complete agreement. The stakes were too high to leave any room for error.

After two hours, Kay and I were allowed to visit briefly with Tracey. He was uncomfortable and nervous. We massaged his hands and feet, and he began to relax. Finally, at 8:30 P.M., the actual radiation began. Tracey would be wide awake during the procedure. There would not be any discomfort or pain, but he would be totally alone. Since no one could be physically in the room, a TV monitor allowed the technicians to watch. I was in an adjacent room, but I felt like I was a million miles away. I prayed. Twenty-five minutes later, a nurse appeared and announced, "It's over. It was successful. You'll be able to see Tracey as soon as the halo is removed."

As I entered, Tracey was sitting up and talking with the nurse as she cleansed and covered the skin where the screws had been inserted. After I kissed him and made sure that he was okay, I felt the adrenaline in the room. There was some conversation, but there were silent high fives going on all around us. It had been very tense, but now everyone was feeling a natural high. Families generally don't have the opportunity to share this experience. It was extraordinary. As I thought about all the years of training, research, and education that the people in this room represented, I was extremely grateful. The only way that I could show our appreciation was to approach each individual, shake their hand, and personally thank them for their help. By the looks on their faces, I could tell that this was highly unusual and unexpected. At first they seemed confused, then embarrassed, and finally appreciative. They were definitely excited by what they had just been able to accomplish.

Apparently, the halo had recently been designed using a lightweight material. Kost was proud of this new device, and I started to chuckle as I watched him. He was just like any other man with a new toy. He wanted to show me. "Take a look at this. See how light it is!" As he handed it to me, I couldn't help myself. I startled him as I cried, "OOPS!" and acted like I was going to drop this very expensive piece of equipment. His face dropped and he protectively removed the halo from my grasp. I very seriously agreed that it was indeed as light as a feather and inquired, "What's it made of?" Realizing that I was having fun at his expense, he smiled and replied, "Graphite." I wasn't quite done poking fun, and said, "Who would have thought that my ski poles would be made of the same material!"

Everyone was coming down from the emotional rush, and fatigue was settling over us all. The ambulance crew was ready to take us back to the hospital. As we were walking out, everyone said, "Good-night." It was almost 9:30 P.M. Kost remarked, "It's been a long day." I nodded and said, "Yes, it has been a long day. Thanks for everything."

As soon as we were settled in the ambulance, Tracey tried to get the driver to use the siren so that we could get back to the main campus of Henry Ford as soon as possible. He was starved. One of the many things Tracey and I had in common was that if we were hungry, we were very cranky. Neither one of us had eaten since lunch. I had packed a dinner, but it was in my car. When Tracey discovered that I had not brought the food, we would not have wanted to be photographed. It was not a pretty picture. Since there was nothing to eat, we bit our tongues and had the good sense to be silent.

By the time Tracey was settled in his bed, he was beyond cranky; he was mad as a hornet. His catheter had leaked and his pants were soaked in urine. Before I had a chance to ring for help, he started to rip at his clothes. I was afraid he was going to pull out his catheter. As soon as the nurse changed his clothes, I started to shovel food in his mouth. Within ten minutes, he calmed down. At about 10:30 P.M., he finished eating and closed his eyes. This had been a traumatic day. We needed to hold each other's hands, so I stayed for another hour. I couldn't leave until he was ready to sleep. As long as there were no complications, Tracey would be discharged tomorrow. Everyone hoped the new tumor site had been eradicated. Only time would tell.

Chapter Fourteen

Remember Rule #1

(Ask your friends and family for help!)

On Friday of Memorial Day weekend, 1995, we were on our way home. Tracey's appearance was deceiving. You would never have known that he had undergone major surgery. He looked and felt fine, but he needed to rest. When he was discharged, there were only two prescriptions. One was Dilantin, to prevent seizures, and the other was Decadron, a steroid to reduce brain swelling. They were beneficial, but Tracey had already experienced the side effects of long term use of prescription drugs. He would be glad when he was weaned off Decadron in two weeks, because at the end of June he was scheduled to begin a new chemotherapy protocol, VP-16.

In the meantime, we were going to enjoy this short reprieve. We started to make plans for all the things we wanted to do during the next six months. Anticipating the future was extremely important. Tracey knew that he wasn't ready yet, but he was determined to water-ski by the end of the summer. Some people thought he was crazy, but this goal gave him a reason to fight and to continue working hard at therapy. Keeping a positive attitude would have been impossible if there were no dreams that could come true. Fun had to remain an integral part of our lives.

We were especially looking forward to a family gathering. Twenty family members were going on a five day cruise to

Mexico in December. My parents were celebrating their fiftieth wedding anniversary. Everyone lived in different parts of the United States; it would be the first time in ten years that we would all be together. Since there was not a lot of preparation to do, it would be a perfect vacation. Everyone was excited.

Although a home care aide was with him while I was at work, Tracey rarely went anywhere except physical therapy. Despite his determination, he was becoming weaker and couldn't walk, even a few steps, unless someone physically supported him. To make matters worse, he had few visitors. As a result, Tracey was becoming isolated. I realized that for three months, he had not gone out with just the guys. I discovered the problem was that his friends were afraid that they would hurt him. They had seen me maneuver around the house with Tracey. Although they were very strong, their attempts to walk with Tracey were awkward and laborious. The finesse that Tracey and I had developed was missing. I showed them some techniques that we found helpful. Gradually, they became confident and planned a house party. The Detroit Red Wings had won a playoff berth. It was the perfect excuse for a boys' night out. In order to avoid any awkwardness, I explained to his buddies that in addition to walking to the bathroom, Tracey would need help pulling down his pants, sitting down on the toilet seat, and cleaning himself when he was finished. Without a moment's hesitation, they replied, "No problem. What are friends for!" None of these men had previous experience helping anyone in this way. I was amazed by the depth of their friendship.

Everything was set. To make things a little easier, I dropped Tracey off at Tim's house. I was like a nervous mother leaving her new baby for the first time. They pushed me out the door and told me not to wait up. At midnight, Tracey came home and was ecstatic. I wasn't a big hockey fan, but Tracey had a story to tell. "The game was tied and the Wings went into triple overtime. Everyone was on the edge of their seat watching the game. You could have cut the tension with a knife. Suddenly, I realized that I had to go to the bathroom. Everyone volunteered to help. In record time, they helped me sit on the toilet and left to give me some privacy. I finished what I had to do and started to call out, 'Guys! Hey guys! I'm done. Guys, come get me!' Unfortunately, their voices were getting louder and louder. Then, they were screaming and I heard high fives. In a few minutes, things quieted down and I heard someone say, 'Where's Tracey?' In all the excitement, they had forgotten all about me. Suddenly, five faces appeared in the doorway of the bathroom and saw a dejected fan sitting on the can. I had missed the winning goal."

In spite of his absence from the highlight of the game, this was a wonderful evening that enabled Tracey and his friends to reconnect. Even though he could not have been happier, Tracey's eyes began to fill with tears. He had become very emotional over the past few months, but I couldn't imagine what was wrong. Maybe he was tired. He wiped away his tears and explained, "I thought that my friends would never want to do anything with me again." Now both of us were crying. Only this time, I knew they were tears of happiness.

Five days after radiosurgery, a miracle happened. Tracey's peripheral vision returned and his balance improved dramatically. He sensed the improvement, and his therapists were amazed by his sudden progress. Our hope was revitalized.

Unfortunately, our excitement was short lived. As quickly as he had started to improve, Tracey's strength and balance disappeared. One morning, I helped him to the bathroom and went to our bedroom. Suddenly, I heard a crash and then complete silence. I rushed to see what had happened. Tracey had fallen off the toilet. Apparently, he had lost his balance as he leaned over to squash a spider that was crawling on the floor. Fortunately, he was only bruised. He wasn't bleeding, and there were no broken bones. However, we were both shaken. I made him promise that there would not be any more big game hunting in the bathroom. Eliminating the spider population in our house was not a priority. Next time, he might end up with a concussion.

While struggling to help him stand, I realized that he could not be left alone in the bathroom. Naturally, I was concerned about his safety. However, I was more afraid that the loss of independence and privacy would be devastating. Tracey had to keep his pride. I needed to be sensitive and allow him to decide how to handle this problem. Thankfully, he wanted someone close by when he was using the bathroom. After all, he didn't want to fall. Next, we tried to figure out why he was tipsy. I remembered that his Decadron dose had been reduced and I left a message for his neurologist. When he returned my call, Tom Mikkelsen said that the loss of balance was probably due to postoperative swelling in the brain. It was not unexpected. The solution was to continue administering Decadron at a higher level for a few weeks. After Tracey was stable, it could be decreased.

The changes that were occurring were very disturbing. Every time he took one step forward, it seemed as if he took five steps backward. It was very disheartening. I knew that his therapists were concerned. Tracey had become more than a patient. He was their friend, and they wanted him to recover. I didn't realize how emotionally attached they had become until Colleen, his occupational therapist, related a story to me.

Every few weeks, Colleen looked forward to meeting a group of friends for dinner. This particular night, they were sitting at a round table and no one was in a good mood. One friend exclaimed that this had been the worst week of her life. Everyone took their turn, and each story seemed worse than the previous one. Finally, it was Colleen's turn. She sighed and without skipping a beat seriously remarked, "My patient fell off the toilet today!" Conversation ceased for a brief moment, jaws dropped, and then everyone burst out laughing. Their troubles suddenly seemed insignificant, and no more complaints were heard that evening.

By the second week of June, Tracey was struggling more every day. His determination and the expertise of his therapists were not making a difference. In order to extend therapy, there had to be progress and achievable goals. The insurance company required a written report from Tracey's therapists every month. It was getting to the point that there was nothing more that they could recommend. Colleen, Lizzy and Ruth were concerned. I crossed my fingers and hoped that increasing Decadron would make a difference.

Gradually, Tracey's balance improved, but his strength and endurance varied from day to day. I was discouraged, exhausted, and angry. Nothing seemed to be going right, and neither of us was getting any sleep. Tracey was getting up at least four times every night to urinate. We had tried three different types of condom catheters. Some easily slipped off during the night. Others had too much adhesive. In the morning, as I gently tried to remove the condom, some of Tracey's skin peeled off with the latex. I tried using adhesive remover. It worked, but there was an obvious problem. Tracey began to scream, "It feels like my balls are on fire!" The remover was alcohol-based and it burned his sensitive skin. We had reached the end of the road as far as condom catheters were concerned. Being pulled, pinched, and peeled was one thing, but Tracey's patience evaporated after his disastrous trial by fire. Although I had not given up hope of finding a solution to this dilemma, I realized that we needed help. Home care during the day was not enough. I couldn't be Superwoman anymore. Something had to give, and it did.

On Sunday, June 11, we went to a graduation party. We hadn't gone anywhere for awhile and were looking forward to seeing our friends. It was not a particularly good day for Tracey, because he was having difficulty walking. When we reached the doorstep of our friend's home, there wasn't a railing that he could use for support. I was trying to lift his left leg when someone volunteered to help. Before I had a chance to give directions, his weight shifted toward my left shoulder. Everyone within a two block radius knew that I was hurt. My shoulder was dislocated again. Our friend, Paul, carried Tracey into the living room. After I was led to the bedroom, I 'adjusted' my shoulder, and it slipped back into place. I was on the brink of having a nervous breakdown and repeatedly sobbed, "I can't do this anymore! I can't do this anymore!" I was an emotional wreck. My mind raced. "What are we going to do? I can't help Tracey walk any more. It isn't safe for either one of us. We need help twenty-four hours a day. How can we afford this new expense?" I didn't have any answers. I wanted someone else to take charge, to save Tracey—to rescue me! I couldn't do it anymore! Just then our friend John, who had given Tracey and me such good advice over the past two years, walked into the room. Once he knew that my shoulder was in place, he held my hand and began talking, "I don't know how you are doing it, Kathy. What can we do? You can't take care of Tracey by yourself anymore. You need help. It's time for you to let your friends help you." I was sobbing and could only nod. He continued, "Tracey has been very worried about you for a long time. You need to find full-time help. Why don't you ask friends to spend the night? They can help Tracey if he needs it." I could hardly speak. Thinking was impossible. I needed rest. John could see that I was exhausted and suggested, "Go to our house where it's quiet. We'll help Tracey. You get some sleep." I went to the living room and told Tracey that I was fine. His eyes were worried, and there was guilt written across his face. He felt like this was all his fault. I kissed him and said, "It's nobody's fault. It was an accident. I'll be fine after I take a nap." Two hours later, I woke up and called Tracey's sister, Claudia. "Can you spend the night? I dislocated my shoulder." As I called our friends, I realized they had wanted to help for a long time but did not know what they could do. Within two hours, I had contacted fourteen friends who could spend the night. I felt like things were under control again. Claudia met us at home that evening and the next morning she helped Tracey dress and drove him to therapy.

Now, I needed to talk with Tracey's doctors. I left emotional voice mail messages telling them that I wanted to discuss the course of treatment they had planned. I wasn't sure that chemotherapy was a viable option anymore. Tracey was deteriorating, and we needed a reality check.

Meanwhile, I needed to take care of myself. Dr. McTurk, our internist, agreed to see me immediately. After he examined and x-rayed my shoulder, he recommended that I see an orthopedic surgeon. Most specialists are scheduled weeks in advance, but I couldn't wait three weeks for an appointment. If surgery was not necessary, I needed a prescription to begin physical therapy as soon as possible. Remembering RULE #1, I contacted Ardis Gregory, who had arranged our appointment with Kost two years ago. She was able to schedule an appointment with a specialist at Henry Ford for Friday at 11 A.M.

When I returned home, there was a message from Tom Mikkelsen on our answering machine. I dialed his number and luckily, he was at his desk. He was worried about both of us and wanted to know what had happened. I quickly summarized what had occurred and took a deep breath, "Tracey is so weak. I don't see how he can tolerate another session of chemo. The quality of his life is very important. If treatment is not working, maybe we should stop." Tom replied without hesitation, "We are by no means at the end of the road. I understand that you are concerned. We need to talk in person. Can you come in?" We arranged to meet on Friday before I saw the orthopedic surgeon.

For two days, I stayed home to rest. I knew that the help we received from friends and family could only be a temporary measure. Tracey's dad, George, had been driving Tracey to physical therapy and visiting while I was at work. However, George was retired and couldn't physically or emotionally be Tracey's caregiver. I discovered that insurance would pay for Tracey's care only if he moved to a nursing facility or was diagnosed as terminal with less than six months to live. Full-time care at home was not a benefit. It made no sense, but those were the rules. There had to be a solution. Suddenly, I had a brainstorm. My cousin, Matt, and my brother, Denis, had careers in education. Since they were on summer vacation, maybe they could help. Without hesitating, they both agreed. Matt lived in Oregon and could arrive by June 30. Denis lived in Tennessee and could stay for two weeks in July. I was relieved. Tracey would be safe, I could continue to work, and we wouldn't have strangers living with us. In the meantime, Peggy, the home care aide, continued to stay with Tracey during the day and friends spent the night.

When I returned to work, my co-workers were incredulous that I had hurt myself. I had a reputation for sports accidents, and every year I was disabled by another injury. Friends saw my sling and simply shook their heads, "What did you do now?" I decided to be a little creative about my bad luck and seriously explained, "I was swinging on our trapeze in the bedroom . . ." Their voices echoed, "A trapeze in the bedroom, you've got to be kidding." After a moment, they realized that I was yanking their chain. We laughed, but no one dared ask me for details twice.

By Friday, I felt more in control. I made a decision not to tell Tracey about my appointment with Dr. Mikkelsen. I needed to have a blunt conversation and did not feel that I would be able to ask all my questions if Tracey were with me. Either this meeting would rekindle my hope, or I would have to plan for what future Tracey and I had left. Tracey would be the final decision-maker regarding chemotherapy, but we both had to feel that it had value. One person could not face this alone. We needed a united front. I could not have any doubts, because Tracey would immediately know.

Tom Mikkelsen greeted me and showed me to his office. After exchanging a few pleasantries, I repeated my concerns and tried to hold back my tears. Tom reassured me, "It's okay to cry. How do you feel about Tracey's progress so far?" I paused for a moment to gather my thoughts. "Tracey does not seem to be getting any better. In fact, every couple of weeks he gets weaker and loses more strength. We have repeatedly said that the quality of life is very important to Tracey. Chemo and surgery have taken their toll. Because his stamina is very low, I'm not sure he can tolerate another session of chemotherapy. He needs to be able to use what little energy he has to enjoy himself while he can. I feel like we are only trying to maintain the quality of his life for as long as we can." I hesitated for a moment and then asked the question that had been on my mind for a very long time but I had been unable to voice, "How much time does Tracey have?" My eyes were locked on Tom's. Thankfully, he did not look away, nor did he beat around the bush. If he had done either of those things, I would not have believed what he said. "I know this is not what you want to hear, but I can't give you a date. Since I have been proven wrong so many times, I have learned not to give predictions. What I can tell you is that I am listening to what you are saying about the quality of life. I feel that VP-16 is beneficial. If the time comes that we feel that treatment is not of value, we will let you know. By the end of July, we should know if the chemotherapy is working. At that time, if the tumor is still growing, Tracey will only have months to live." I knew that this was not an easy conversation for either one of us, and I could see Tom was genuinely concerned and understood my sorrow. I felt like a huge burden had been lifted from my shoulders. I knew that I was not alone. There is a saying, "The truth will set you free." I was now free to react to the information I had received. I chose to be hopeful, for myself as well as Tracey. We still had time to enjoy life together.

I had one remaining question, but it was not about Tracey. It was about Tom. "Do you mind if I ask you something? How did you get into this specialty? Most of your patients die. I don't know how you do it." He smiled and said, "There are two reasons. First, the scientific research interests me. Second, most terminal patients are short-changed. In order to protect themselves, many physicians build walls between themselves and their patients. Terminal patients deserve better. They deserve the best." I nodded in agreement and thought, "Tracey does have the best doctors. We are very lucky."

There are many points of view regarding communication with cancer patients. I think every person needs to be treated as an individual. There are no cookie cutter answers. During the course of his illness, hope enabled Tracey to survive. His physicians protected him by not using words like "cancer," "malignant," and "terminal." They are only words, but their impact is destructive to the human spirit. They imply death. Tracey needed to be positive and look forward to the future. In order to continue his battle, he had to feel he had a chance to live. He did not need to have anyone remind him that he could die. Every day when he looked in the mirror, he could not escape the horrible truth—his body was failing.

I headed for my appointment with the orthopedic surgeon. After he reviewed my case history, he examined my shoulder and found that I had significant strength and flexibility. The surgeon recommended physical therapy for six weeks. I was relieved, but now I had to juggle our schedule and squeeze another set of appointments into our calendar. Generally, physical therapy must be prearranged three weeks in advance. I took advantage of RULE #1. A friend at work called his sister, who in turned called a friend, who . . . to make a long story short, I had an appointment within a week. Fortunately, Henry Ford had a facility close to my job, and my therapist, Chris, was very flexible. As a result, I was able to work out during my lunch hour twice a week.

I was improving physically by the end of June, but emotionally I was a wreck. I vacillated between being on the verge of crying and exploding in anger. Rage boiled just below the surface. I realized that I needed professional help. Thankfully, my insurance benefits provided the means to obtain immediate counseling. Over a four-week period, a psychologist gave me practical suggestions on how to solve problems and open communication with our families. These sessions allowed me to grieve openly and share my anguish—in confidence—with someone who was totally impartial. Gradually, my feelings of control increased, and my frustration level declined. I didn't want to put my emotional health in jeopardy. Whenever I became upset, I was able to regain my perspective by taking a deep breath. My creed became, "Don't worry about the things you can't control." I refused to waste my energy harboring any anger. As my inner strength improved, a sense of calmness returned to our lives.

Meanwhile, Tracey was holding his own. He wasn't making any significant gains, but he wasn't losing ground either. Having friends spend the night had two advantages. First, Tracey was safe moving around the house. Second, it was wonderful having company. Because Tracey retired relatively early, our bedroom became our living room in the evening. We would visit and watch television, and Tracey could drift off to sleep. Before long, we felt that our company was really part of our family.

Life was much less stressful, but Tracey and I were still not getting a good night's sleep. It seemed like every time I drifted off, Tracey would wake me because he needed to urinate. I found a solution in the most unlikely of places. Once a month for five years, I had been having dinner with a group of women. At times, they had become my sounding board and offered help when they could. One friend, Colleen, had a sister who sold medical equipment to urologists. Her sister talked to a pharmacist who suggested something called a "sheath urinal." After telephoning the pharmacist, I decided to drive forty minutes and see how this urinal worked. The pharmacist was very understanding and listened attentively to my tale of woe. Before I actually saw the apparatus, we talked for thirty minutes.

There were three sizes—small, medium, and large. He wanted to know, "What size will your husband need?" I was amused, and was tempted to say extra large, but instead suggested, "Let's try medium to start." He pulled a box off the shelf. Inside there was a jock strap and a hollow rubber penis which could hold about five fluid ounces. On its tip, there was a removable cap which could be unscrewed. It was very difficult to keep a straight face as he gave me directions. "First, align the snaps and attach the urinal (rubber penis) to the jock strap. Your husband will need to put on the jock strap and insert his penis into the rubber sheath. In order to prevent urine from leaking, the rubber sheath will fit snugly around the shaft of his penis. After unscrewing the cap, the urinal can be attached to a foley bag which you can drain in the morning." This appeared simple enough. If it worked, we would have our first good night's sleep in over two months.

I rushed home and showed Tracey. We both laughed at what became affectionately known as Big Bad Joe. He was ready to try anything, as long as it didn't feel like his balls were on fire. That evening, our first attempts were very awkward. Since Tracey couldn't use his left hand, putting on Joe had to be a joint effort. After stretching, pushing, and pulling for what seemed like an eternity, everything looked secure. We crossed our fingers and went to sleep. At about 1 A.M., Tracey nudged me, "I have to pee!" I threw back the sheets to see if Joe worked. Two minutes later, you would have thought we had successfully launched the first space shuttle. Our mission was accomplished without any casualties. Joe was our new best friend.

It's amazing how a night of uninterrupted sleep changes your whole attitude. Tracey and I both began to have new energy and optimism. By the end of June, we had a new lease on life. Adventure, laughter, and fun appeared on our doorstep with the arrival of my cousin, Matt.

Chapter Fifteen

Sharing Love, Laughter, and Prized Possessions

On Thursday, June 29, 1995, I was rushing home from work. If I was fifteen minutes late, I would lose four hours of home care. As I pulled into our driveway, an unfamiliar station wagon was parked in my spot. I was irritated until I noticed the Oregon license plates; Matt had arrived a day early. When I walked into the house, two smiling faces greeted me. Tracey and Matt were like two Cheshire cats who had swallowed the family parakeet. They proudly announced, "We've been very busy fixing dinner. Hurry up and change your clothes. Nobody likes cold food." I don't recall what we ate that evening, but I do remember feeling terribly thankful. Being surprised with dinner was great, however, it was wonderful to see Tracey's eyes sparkling. It had been a long time since he had been able to take care of me. He was constantly worried that he was taking advantage of me. Love is a two-way street, and he needed to give as well as receive.

Life became much less complicated for me. I didn't need to worry about scheduling friends and family to help transport Tracey to therapy or chemo. Thankfully, we could delay using the remaining 'home care allotment' until September. Most importantly, Tracey was safe. Matt became Tracey's constant companion and his friend. During the day, Tracey now had a life. He was able to go places, see people and do things. In order to help me, they decided to do all the grocery shopping. Going to the supermarket became an adventure.

One day, Tracey and Matt decided to go to Meijer Thrifty Acres, a superstore, where everything you could possibly want was under one roof. By the time they parked and walked to the entrance, Tracey was exhausted. Matt decided to go back to the car and get Tracey's wheelchair. They were trying to find a place for Tracey to wait when a store hostess approached them. "Would you like to use one of our motorized carts?" This appeared to be the perfect solution. Operating instructions seemed simple enough. Steering the cart was just like a bike; the brakes and power were activated by controls on the handlebar. Tracey took off. He was enjoying this new independence. Just like a race track, the straightaway was not a problem, but curves proved to be dangerous. Since Tracey could only use his right arm, turning, accelerating, and simultaneously braking were treacherous. As he was learning to navigate, a pyramid of lettuce became a casualty and tumbled to the floor. A clerk asked Tracey if he was okay and rebuilt the display without another word. Tracey thought they would revoke his privilege to drive, so he made a hasty retreat from the produce department. There were a few near collisions, but nothing more was demolished. On the way out, the hostess asked Tracey if he wanted to drive the cart to his car. He laughed, "I'm dangerous enough in the store. I don't think the outside world is ready for me yet."

Although Tracey was having difficulty walking, it was fairly easy to use our pontoon boat. However, boarding our ski boat was another matter. As long as three people helped, he was able to step from the dock to the ski platform and into the boat. Neither one of us was going to water-ski this summer, but we wanted to enjoy the water. We planned on taking our friends tubing and water-skiing. In July, the temperatures soared to new highs. In order to escape the heat, we went for boat rides and occasionally swam in the lake. One day, Tracey put on a life vest and began to eye the inner-tube. "Do you think I could go tubing?" Without hesitating, I said, "Of course!" Since the tube had a bottom, he could safely sit in the middle. As he floated away, the rope became taut. Tracey gave me the thumbs up, and I put the boat in gear. To my horror, Tracey began to sink. His body weight was on the wrong side of the tube. We quickly pulled him back to the boat and tried to reposition him. Suddenly, I started to scream. My shoulder was dislocated. Within seconds, I popped it back in place and joked, "If I didn't have bad luck, I wouldn't have any at all!" Since I wasn't in any pain, everyone agreed that Tracey should still tube. Matt and my cousin Patti pushed the tube away from the boat, and I drove. As we gained speed, Tracey's eyes were round as saucers. However, the smile on his face disappeared when he hit some waves from another watercraft. He immediately signaled that he was done. As we pulled him into the boat he whispered, "That was fun but I don't think I want to try it again for awhile."

One of Matt and Tracey's favorite field trips was going to buy fresh coffee beans at a store that had a frequent shopper program. After purchasing ten pounds of coffee, they received one pound free. Since our freezer was packed with over fifteen different flavors, it seemed to me that Tracey and Matt had received more than their fair share of free coffee. I'm not sure if they confused the clerk or flirted with her, but they made out like bandits. Every morning, there was a major decision to make. "Do we want Mackinaw Chocolate Fudge or Hot Butter Rum? Maybe a Kona blend would be better!" They both loved coffee, and now it was an obsession. Although I did not care to become a coffee connoisseur, I learned to recognize the distinct aromas of the various blends.

As they sipped their morning brew, Tracey developed another hobby: birdwatching. The dining room windows faced our backyard, and Matt and Tracey decided it was the perfect place to observe birds. Since they wanted to attract as many varieties as possible, they erected four feeders and filled them with gourmet seed. Nothing but the best for their fair-feathered friends. For three days, they watched and waited. Finally, on the fourth day, a blue jay discovered pay dirt. By the end of the second week, our yard looked like a scene from Alfred Hitchcock's movie, *The Birds*. Luckily, the birds never attacked us, but they did make a racket. Then, the inevitable happened—a squirrel staked its claim. Now it became a battle of man against beast. Matt and Tracey plotted and planned their strategy to fight this unwelcome invasion. Since every feeder was designed differently, they spent the rest of the summer trying to defeat this cunning opponent by creating temporary roadblocks. While the squirrel developed new tactics, flocks of birds descended. It was only a matter of time before the foul odor from their poop forced us to close our windows. One day, I was talking to our next door neighbor, Linda, about our bird stench. She casually suggested that we might want to consider moving the feeders away from our air conditioning unit. As I walked to the side of our house, I noticed that it looked like someone had gone crazy painting white dots on our neighbor's new brick sidewalk. Reality settled in and I was mortified. Linda didn't want to complain, and said, "We leave early in the morning and come home late at night. It's always so dark, we barely notice." But our birds were a menace. After a brief discussion, Tracey and Matt decided it was a good idea to halt the feeding frenzy and eliminate two of the feeders. Our neighbors were good friends, and we wanted to keep it that way.

During the day, life was settling into a routine. By the time I came home in the evening, Matt was exhausted. Helping Tracey was more than one person could handle. Even though he was not confined to a wheelchair, Tracey could not walk anywhere by himself. He had to rely on us to help him stand up and sit down, as well as walk from room to room. Since he needed to urinate at least once an hour, it was very difficult to leave Tracey alone for more than five minutes at a time. Even when he took a nap, someone had to be close. We unsuccessfully tried using a bell and a whistle. Finally, Linda gave me the wonderful suggestion of a baby monitor. It enabled Tracey to communicate with us when we were not within earshot, it gave us some measure of freedom to move around the house, and Tracey felt safe. It was the perfect solution.

Toward the middle of July, my brother Denis arrived. We were beginning to feel housebound and decided that it was time to plan a weekend trip. Matt's parents had invited us to visit them in Ontario, Canada. For over thirty-five years, my family had gathered at the cottage during summers and holidays. I joked that we were the only family I knew who drove three hours in order to take naps and eat. Mealtime was an event, because frequently there were over twenty mouths to feed. Many times, five conversations were occurring simultaneously—that is until food was served. As soon as we finished saying grace, the only noise was the clatter of silverware as the various dishes were passed. Everyone knew if they weren't careful, they could easily starve. During the rest of the day, keeping busy was not a problem. We entertained ourselves by sunbathing on the beach, swimming in Lake Huron, reading books, walking to town, and playing games. It could be very peaceful, however, at any moment a cutthroat game of cards could erupt. If we had one thing in common, it was our competitive nature. No matter what the age, three or eighty, we all wanted to win. I hate to admit it, but I personally had a hard time letting even a child win at checkers. My rationalization for this strange behavior was, "You can't expect to win all the time. Children need to learn how to lose too." However, I was outsmarted by my seven year old cousin, Jaime. We were playing a card game that seemed like it would never end. No matter how hard I tried to allow Jaime to win, she kept losing. Finally, I realized she didn't care about winning. She just wanted to continue playing cards, and knew the game would be over if she won. Jaime had a captive playmate and would not let me surrender gracefully. Fortunately, dinner was served an hour later and I was saved.

The cottage had always been a retreat from the outside world, but spending time there also gave us the opportunity to strengthen our family ties. Everyone was aware that Tracey was seriously ill and might not recover. Although only the adults had the physical strength to help him move, the children were the ones who lifted Tracey's spirits. They were sensitive to his needs, and often offered to fluff a pillow or bring him something to drink. They were not afraid to touch or talk with Tracey and he was able to enjoy their laughter as they played nearby. Unlike adults, their eyes did not reflect fear or sadness. They shone with love and concern.

It has been my observation that frequently, children are not allowed to participate in the care of someone who may die. A parent's rationalization may be that they are trying to protect their children from the tragedy of death. However, instead of allowing their children to learn how to embrace life, they are teaching fear and preventing them from sharing their love. This is not to imply that children do not need guidance and support. Unfortunately, many adults have very few coping skills themselves, let alone the experience to counsel anyone else. Professional help is available, but I discovered a wonderful book by Elisabeth Kubler-Ross, M.D., entitled *Death is of Vital Importance*. Not only does it give practical suggestions for talking about death with children, but it was also very helpful to me, as Tracey's health was steadily declining.

After our weekend getaway, we returned home. Matt needed a break and remained in Canada. Luckily, my brother Denis was able to stay with us for a week. As we approached the Detroit area, there was a severe weather alert. Heavy winds pushed ominous black clouds across the sky, and lightning began to flash across the horizon. Suddenly, the heavens opened and sheets of rain pounded the car. The storm subsided when we pulled into the driveway. We were able to walk into the house without getting soaked, but discovered that there was a power outage. In a few moments, the downpour continued; the backyard became saturated. When the rain finally stopped, there were four inches of standing water in our driveway. Since there was no electricity, the sump pump was out of commission, and our lower level flooded. There were three inches of water in the utility room, and the carpet in the family room was a soaked sponge. Nothing was draining, so the bucket brigade went into action. Denis and I bailed over seventy gallons of water from the basement into the lake. Finally, it seemed that things were under control, and we stopped for dinner. Unfortunately, thirty minutes later it looked like we hadn't removed any water, and we decided to move all the furniture upstairs. By the time we were done, we were exhausted and went to bed. At 7 A.M. the next morning, there still wasn't any electricity. Denis took Tracey to physical therapy, and I rented a generator. By 10 A.M., the sump pump had drained all the standing water, and I was able to begin cleaning up the mess. At 4 P.M., power was back to normal. But for three days, Denis used a wet/dry home-n-shop vac in an attempt to salvage our carpet. In addition, we borrowed heavy-duty fans, and bought an extra dehumidifier to help decrease the moisture. Once everything was dry, Tracey's dad was able to retack the carpet and a week later, everything was back in place. We had been very lucky and had escaped with very little damage. However, it seemed that every time I felt like things were finally under control, something happened to upset the apple cart. It was hard enough handling the ups and downs of Tracey's illness, but Mother Nature had come knocking at our door. If it had not been for the support of our families, I would have had a nervous breakdown.

At the beginning of July, Tracey underwent yet another type of chemo. By the middle of the month, he was totally exhausted. It had become a real struggle even to get to physical therapy. His physical stamina was very low and his physiatrist, Dr. Sesi, suggested taking a break from therapy for six weeks. Tracey accepted this bad news stoically. I cried. Even though it was possible to start therapy again at a later time, my gut told me that no matter what we did, cancer was winning. Another crossroads was quickly approaching. Tracey was scheduled for his first CAT scan since the radiosurgery in May. During the week we waited for the results, I held my breath. I wanted to know the outcome, but at the same time I didn't want to know. When we met with Tracey's neurosurgeon at the end of July, we tried to brace ourselves for bad news. Kost did not waste any time. "The CAT scan looks good. There hasn't been any significant tumor growth." We were both relieved, but I was still concerned. During the exam, I mentioned some subtle changes that I had noticed. Tracey's speech was slightly slurred, and his short term memory was getting worse. Kost accepted my observations but said, "I can't detect any major problems. Tracey seems to be doing well." I started to become upset, because I felt like I was being ignored. Then, Kost briefly looked in my direction and his eyes spoke what he could not say, "Tracey needs hope." My impatience slipped away, and I refocused on the good news we had just received. "The CAT scan looks good."

The following week, Tracey was scheduled to begin another cycle of chemo. Dr. Wollner arranged his schedule so that we could meet with him after our appointment with the neurosurgeon. All of Tracey's physicians understood the problems associated with trying to consult five different specialists. I was working full-time and needed to coordinate doctor visits as much as possible. Even though these physicians were very busy, they always attempted to be flexible in order to help us. During our meeting with Dr. Wollner, he reviewed Tracey's bloodcounts, which had dropped dangerously low. During the eighteen months that Tracey had received chemo, this had never happened. The next dosage of chemo would be adjusted so that Tracey would not be so exhausted. As we left Henry Ford Medical Center, we breathed a sigh of relief, because we had a six week reprieve before the next doctor's appointment and CAT scan. We were trying to keep an optimistic attitude.

To the casual observer, it may have appeared that I was in a state of denial regarding Tracey's health, but I was choosing to think and act positively. I continued to try to plan activities that we could enjoy together. On October 6, 1995, we would celebrate our tenth wedding anniversary. I wanted to arrange something special and bought tickets for an Elton John concert, which just happened to be on Friday, October 6. This was going to be a very difficult secret to keep, because Elton John was Tracey's favorite musician. I could hardly wait to surprise him. Another family event was the Mexico cruise in December to celebrate my parents' fiftieth wedding anniversary. In spite of all the setbacks, Tracey and I chose to make plans for the future.

Discussing Tracey's prognosis with Shelley and the rest of Tracey's family was one of the most difficult things I had to do. They all loved Tracey and he loved them. Every time they came to visit, there were new problems. Nothing could prepare them for the changes in Tracey's appearance. Although I worried about these changes on a daily basis, I had become accustomed to accepting them. To a certain extent, I only saw the man I loved. They too saw the man they loved, but he was fading away, and there was nothing they could do. Every visit must have been devastating for them. Sharing my fears and feelings with anyone had always been difficult for me. However, I knew I needed to talk with them. They could see that Tracey's health was deteriorating, but they needed to know that he might only have a few months to live. I decided that I would relate what the neurologist, Tom Mikkelsen, had told me. "If the next CAT scan shows that the tumor is growing, Tracey will only have months to live." I cautioned them that I had made a decision not to share this information with Tracey. He knew that every CAT scan could bring bad news, but he did not need to hear, "He might die!" They may or may not have agreed, but they respected my decision. We all loved Tracey and wanted only what was best for him. They continued to be hopeful.

Evening continued to be our private time. Many times when we turned out the lights, we would talk for an hour before going to sleep. Most often we talked about our day, but sometimes we discussed something that was troubling us. One night we were holding hands and letting the darkness settle over us. It was very quiet until Tracey's voice broke the silence, "Did the doctors tell you that I'm dying?" Without hesitating, I whispered, "No! The doctors have not said that you are dying. What they have said is that they feel there are treatments that they can recommend. They understand that you are willing to fight as long as there is a chance to survive and maintain quality in your life. They told me that when they feel that the chemo is not working, they will tell us." Tracey trusted me. He simply said, "If I'm dying, I don't want to be the last to know." I promised, "You will be the first to know." We kissed one another goodnight. Tracey fell asleep and I prayed for a miracle.

The next few weeks flew by. The end of August was approaching quickly, and Matt would be leaving to return to Oregon. Although Tracey wasn't as tired as he had been, he took a nap every day. During the day, Shelley and Tracey's family frequently visited while I was at work. To escape the heat, they occasionally went to the movies and out to eat. Making plans ahead of time was becoming more difficult, because Tracey never knew how much energy he would have. His best days were when he was surrounded by activity. He especially enjoyed spending time with my cousins' children. They entertained him by playing their musical instruments, swam with him in the lake, and included him in outings. One Saturday, we went to a little league game and watched my twelve year old cousin, Scott, pitch. The following week as I was getting ready for work, Tracey asked me to get one of his prized possessions and put it in his knapsack. I went to the bottom drawer of his dresser and found a scuffed baseball. In the early 1960's, Rocky Colavito had hit a homerun during a Tiger game, and it had landed in Tracey's outstretched mitt. Tracey had held onto this treasure for more than thirty years. As I placed the baseball in his knapsack, he simply said, "I don't need this ball any more, and I thought Scott might like it." I couldn't speak, so I nodded my head and kissed him good-bye. As I drove to work, tears streamed down my face. Tracey was beginning to accept what the rest of us could not. He knew that he was dying.

Chapter Sixteen

One Step at a Time

I was beginning to become nervous. Matt was going back to Oregon in ten days. Finding a reliable home care agency was crucial. My cousins Patti and Barb volunteered to help Tracey every Thursday and Friday. This meant that we would only need an aide three days a week. I called an organization that had been recommended by Tracey's therapists. Although they did not have a contract with Tracey's insurance carrier, they agreed to work with our primary care physician, Dr. McTurk, in order to obtain the appropriate approvals. From previous experience, I knew that Michelle, Dr. McTurk's assistant, was dependable. If anyone could navigate through all the red tape, she would. Within a few days, all paperwork was in order and a representative from the home care agency visited. She evaluated Tracey's specific needs and documented his medical background. I was impressed by her responsiveness and professionalism. Matt suggested that he work with the assigned aide, Mary, for a couple of days. In this way, she could become familiar with our daily routines, and Tracey would not be left alone with a stranger. Mary was very accommodating and pleasant. Without prompting, she volunteered to do laundry and perform light housekeeping, and was willing to prepare dinner in addition to breakfast and lunch. Most importantly, she treated Tracey with compassion and respect. I couldn't believe our good luck.

Finally, Matt's departure day arrived. As I hugged him, tears welled in my eyes, and a lump formed in my throat. "Thank you" did not come close to what I wanted to say. Finally, I whispered, "You saved our lives, Matt. I love you." As Tracey and Matt said their good-byes, I had to turn away. They were trying to be upbeat, and they talked about seeing each other on the cruise in December. They were friends and had their own special way of communicating. During the summer, Tracey had noticed that whenever Matt was momentarily at a loss for words during a conversation, he would pause and then point his index finger up in the air. As I waved good-bye, Tracey smiled, raised his right arm, and pointed his index finger at Matt.

A week passed, and I couldn't help noticing that Tracey was becoming very quiet. Labor Day weekend, I invited our water-skiing friends for brunch. The weather was still warm, so we were able to enjoy each other's company and eat outside. His spirits were a little better, but by 1 P.M. he wanted to go inside and take a nap. His legs were so weak that he needed help from our friends Paul and Mark in order to walk upstairs.

Tracey was not looking forward to the next week. Three days of chemo was scheduled. I decided that he needed something to lift his spirits, so I told him about the Elton John concert. He was definitely excited and my surprise had the desired effect. However, by the end of the week, his strength had diminished even more. Every Friday, my cousin Barb picked Tracey up and they went to a coffee house. I wasn't sure that Tracey would have the energy to leave the house, but he was determined to go out. This was his reward for completing another cycle of chemo. That evening we had dinner with Barb's family. As we were getting ready to go home, Tracey suddenly collapsed. Thankfully, we were able to seat him in his wheelchair before he fell on the floor. His eyes were lifeless and his right side was shaking. I called out his name, but he did not respond. This was not normal. Something was terribly wrong. I was ready to call 911, when Tracey regained consciousness. He had a frightened look on his face and asked, "What happened? I could hear you talking but I couldn't say anything." This was the first time that Tracey experienced a seizure. It lasted only two or three minutes. Even though we had been warned that this could happen, it scared me. I tried to remain calm and reassure Tracey. I immediately phoned the neurologist on call and was told that since Tracey was coherent, nothing could be done. At this point, I should watch him closely. He would probably be very tired, but as long as nothing changed, I should notify his physician on Monday. There was a time when I would have wanted immediate answers, but I had gradually discovered over the past two years that many times there were no answers. You just had to wait and see.

When we arrived home, Tracey used what remaining strength he had to climb the stairs and fall into bed. Over the next two days, there were no more problems. We both rested. When I talked to Tom Mikkelsen on Monday, he wanted to have some blood tests performed. As long as Tracey wasn't experiencing any more problems, he was not overly concerned. Over the next week, Tracey became weaker and weaker. He was struggling to walk even fifteen feet. Tracey had rarely complained about the home care aides. However, he began to object to how he was being treated—he did not feel safe.

Suddenly, he started to become restless during the night. He tried to be quiet, but he could not fall asleep. Since he couldn't move out of bed by himself, he started wiggling his foot, raising his arms, and pulling at the sheets. At first, I was able to help him relax by helping him stretch his arm and leg. I could feel the tension release, and he dozed off. However, an hour later he would wake up and the anxiety attacks would return. Neither of us was getting any sleep. Without warning, he started to become distressed during the middle of the day. I telephoned his neurologist and reported these new problems. Before recommending any course of action, he wanted to have Tracey's blood tested again to check the level of steroids and seizure medication. After verifying that there was not a drug imbalance, he prescribed a tranquilizer.

Seven days had passed since these symptoms started, and I was suffering from sleep deprivation. Thank God it was the weekend. Maybe I would finally be able to get some rest. As long as I was close by during the day, Tracey was fine, but as soon as I was out of sight, he would become agitated. Nighttime was getting worse. In order to get some sleep, I moved into another bedroom. I slept for what seemed like fifteen minutes when suddenly Tracey cried out, "Help me! Oh, please help me!" I tried everything I could think of, but nothing worked. First thing Saturday morning, I called Henry Ford Hospital and talked to the neurologist on call. He thought that Tracey might be having an allergic reaction, so he prescribed Benadryl. Tracey started to relax when morning arrived, but by sundown he was an emotional wreck. I called the hospital again. This time the physician prescribed a strong sedative. Tracey and I were willing to try anything. Sunday night, neither one of us slept. By Monday morning, Tracey was completely wired and in a constant state of motion.

I was too exhausted to go to work and at 8 A.M., I left a frantic message for Tom Mikkelsen. I related the problems that had occurred over the weekend. Tracey was scheduled for a CAT scan at 6 P.M. Unless they sedated him, he would not be able to lie completely still. Tom's nurse, Sharon, returned my call, and I began to weep. Between sobs, I was able to describe Tracey's symptoms. She felt that we should proceed with the planned CAT scan, but she wanted to talk with Tom. At noon, Sharon called again and said, "You probably won't like this, but we want to admit Tracey to the hospital. We think that he is having seizures. Can you drive here right now?" Tracey was so weak that I was afraid he would fall down the stairs. I looked outside and our neighbor, Jack, was walking down the street. With his help, we were able to walk safely to the car. Otherwise, I would have had to call 911. Before we left the house, I called my cousin Jake; he would meet us at Henry Ford when we arrived. I was a nervous wreck, and I really had to concentrate while I was driving. We did not need to be in a car accident.

By 4 P.M., the admission paperwork was completed, and Tracey was escorted to his room. After he was heavily sedated, the CAT scan was administered without a problem. The results would not be available until the next day. At 10 P.M., Tracey was sleeping soundly, so I decided to leave. By the time I arrived home, I was too exhausted to think or worry. I fell into bed and slept for the first time in over a week.

At 11 A.M. the next morning, I arrived at Tracey's room. He was surrounded by a group of seven people. It was morning rounds. I entered the room and Tom Mikkelsen said, "There she is. I told you that Kathy would be here." When Tracey had awakened, he was very upset because he did not know where I was. He was frightened and did not remember that he had spent the night in the hospital. As I approached, I was like Moses parting the Red Sea; everyone moved away from the hospital bed. No one said a word, but the looks on their faces told me that the results of the CAT scan were not good. I kissed Tracey and followed Tom as he walked toward the door. I was very direct, "Do you have the results?" He solemnly nodded and suggested that I come to his office anytime after 1 P.M. to talk. I didn't want to talk. I wanted to run away. He couldn't tell me anything that I didn't already know.

Tracey ate lunch and immediately fell into a deep sleep. His nurse told me, "Tracey has been very agitated all morning. It is amazing. As soon as you walked in the room, he calmed right down." I was nervous about leaving Tracey alone, but a student nurse agreed to stay until I returned from my meeting with Tom. By now it was 2 P.M. When I reached the Neurosurgery Department, I stood in the hallway and stared out a window for fifteen minutes. How could I face this alone? Did I have enough strength? Delaying any longer would not change the outcome. My legs felt like they were locked in leg irons, but they moved me toward my destination. Tom was working in his office, and I sat in a chair on the other side of his desk. Generally, I have a remarkable memory for details. However, I can remember only fragments of our conversation. Tom confirmed my worst fears. "Both tumors have recurred and are at the point that we cannot recommend any further treatment." Tears streamed down my face, but I did not fall apart. I had expected bad news. What I didn't anticipate was the answer to my next question, "How much time does Tracey have?" There was no way to soften the blow as Tom replied, "One, maybe two months." I felt like I had been slammed against the wall. Had I heard correctly? How could this be happening? I took a deep breath and exhaled. I hadn't been knocked out, but I was steeling myself against the next blow as I asked, "How bad is it going to be? Will Tracey lose his sight? What should I expect?" Tom explained, "Tracey will begin to sleep more and more. Eventually, he will slip into a coma and will die. He won't lose his vision and there will be no pain. I've arranged for a social worker to help you work out the details for hospice." The only thing left to discuss was who would tell Tracey. For two years, I had been breaking bad news to everyone. I didn't want to—no, I couldn't tell Tracey he was dying. Tom volunteered to talk with Tracey at 1 P.M. the next day. We wanted to wait, so that Tracey would be rested. We also made a decision to tell Tracey that he had half a year to live. I felt that the truth would destroy his will to live. I was not ready for him to die. I needed to spend time with my husband.

Since all the details seemed to be arranged, I changed the subject. We talked for about ten minutes. As I rose to leave, Tom came around his desk and we hugged each other. I was emotionally drained. I was able to keep my composure, but knew that I needed to find a lavatory quickly. In the privacy of a bathroom stall, I wept for myself. I was losing the most important person in my life. No matter what I did, love was slipping away from me once again.

The next twenty-four hours were hell. I had promised Tracey, that he would be the first to know that he was dying. It was a terrible secret to keep. I talked to family members on the phone and discouraged all visitors. I explained that Tracey was drugged and wouldn't be himself. Since he would be discharged fairly soon, it would be better if they delayed seeing him. He would be home by Thursday.

I was constantly on the verge of tears. When Tom arrived at 1 P.M. on Wednesday, Tracey was not awake. The new combination of medication was working too well. He was so tired that he only briefly woke up to eat dinner. The hospital staff arranged for a cot so that I could spend the night. At 10 P.M., I turned off the lights and fell asleep. At midnight, the nurses woke Tracey to give him his medication. After they left, Tracey never went back to sleep. By 2 A.M., he was calling for help. He was having another anxiety attack. I didn't know what to do. Medication was not working; maybe activity would help. I convinced his nurses to transfer Tracey to his wheelchair. For the next two hours, we visited every hospital floor. I know that we were probably breaking every rule, but no one interfered or questioned us. At 4 A.M., we paused by a window at the end of a hallway. The view was spectacular. The city lights sparkled in the clear night sky, and under different circumstances, it would have been very romantic. It was very peaceful and Tracey was finally calm. I knelt on the floor next to his wheelchair and wrapped my arms protectively around him. I could not wait any longer. I felt like my heart was breaking as I began speaking the unspeakable, "Tracey, you have been sick for a long time, and you know that things have not been getting any better. The CAT scan showed that your tumors are growing back. Your doctors don't feel that there is anything more that they can do." Tracey quietly whispered, "Oh no." For a few moments, nothing was said. I rested my head on his shoulder and cried. Finally, Tracey broke the silence, "How can I tell Shelley? What about the rest of my family?" He wasn't worried about himself. There was no anger or bitterness. He loved his family and wanted to protect us. I promised, "I'll tell everyone. You don't need to worry. When you see Shelley, your family, and your friends, they will already know. You won't have to tell anyone." I paused for a moment and continued, "I'm going to take a leave of absence from work. You don't have to worry about home care any more. I will make sure that you are safe." He only asked one more question, "How long do I have?" In the darkness of the hallway, I hoped that he could not see my eyes as I said, "Half a year." After a few moments, we talked about our life together and reminisced about the fun and adventures that we had shared. We comforted each other the only way we knew how. We quietly held each other's hands, looked into each other's eyes, and spoke the only words that mattered—"I love you." I could tell that Tracey was tired. He was ready to go to bed—as long as I was with him. When he was settled, I closed the door, turned out the lights, and squeezed into the hospital bed next to my husband. I wrapped my arms around him and gently stroked the side of his face. Within minutes, he was sleeping peacefully.

When we woke the next morning, the sun was shining, and it seemed like a heavy fog had lifted. The tension in the air had evaporated. Breakfast was delivered, and I prepared the tray so Tracey could eat. I'm not sure what I expected to happen once Tracey had been told that he was dying. The world did not come crashing down. Instead, we simply continued to live. Tracey was quietly eating breakfast, and he casually remarked, "You know, I still have a dream that will come true." I was incredulous and asked, "What do you mean, honey?" He smiled and said, "I've always wanted to see Elton John perform, and we have tickets for his concert." Tracey always had a very positive outlook, but this was beyond what I ever could have imagined. At that moment, I vowed to myself, "Yes, we're going to the concert. But somehow, someway, I'm going to make sure that you meet Elton John too!" Remarkably, he continued to make other suggestions. "Maybe in January we could go skiing in Canada." I swallowed my grief and whispered, "Trace, you are very weak now. Do you think that you'll be able to get strong enough to ski?" He digested what I said and with a tinge of disappointment changed the subject. "Who will go with you on the cruise in December?" Tears streamed down my face. I couldn't pretend that we would be going together. I simply shook my head and replied, "Honey, I don't know. I don't think I'll ever be able to find anybody else who will put up with me." Tracey was testing the waters. He knew that he would not survive for six months.

Before Tracey could be discharged, we needed to meet with his doctors. As we met with Tom and Kost, I could tell that this was very difficult for them. We talked for a few minutes, and they told me to call if I needed any help. Mercifully, they did not say good-bye. They simply said, "Take care." Later, a routine exam was performed by a staff physician. He apologized, but he needed to ask Tracey a few questions. I thought to myself, "Here we go again! Another test to pass." However, this time there were only three questions. First, "Where are you?" Easy answer: "Henry Ford Hospital." Second, "What month is it?" Tracey looked worried and said, "February?" Third, "What is the year?" He replied, "1994." I must have gasped because the doctor looked in my direction. I covered my lips with my fingers, and was trying to hold back the tears. It was Thursday, September 21, 1995. How could I have been so blind? I had no idea how bad Tracey's memory was. The man I loved was fading away.

By the time Tracey was finally discharged, it was 3 P.M. When we were about ten minutes from the house, Tracey began to have a panic attack. He had been fine the entire day. I couldn't figure out what was wrong. Tracey couldn't explain why he was becoming agitated. My cousin Patti met us at our doorway. Once we were inside, Tracey painstakingly climbed the stairway, one step at a time. As soon as he lay down in bed, his anxiety disappeared. He had been afraid. He looked at me and sighed, "I don't want to go on the stairs again."

We were home to stay.

Chapter Seventeen

Can You Feel the Love Tonight?

Now that we were home, I had to keep my next promise—I had to tell everyone else that Tracey was dying. I tried to plan what I would say. I needed to find the right words, but there were none. In three hours, Shelley would arrive. I had called Shelley's mom, Connie, and asked her to come too. Shelley would need the love of her mother.

I also knew that I needed help at night. I had called our friends, and different people agreed to spend the next four nights. Others offered to bring meals. Tonight, Don and Diane would stay with us.

At 7 P.M., Shelley and Connie arrived. I asked Don and Diane to keep Tracey company while I talked with them. How do you tell a child that her father is going to die? How do you soften the blow? The facts were too harsh. I could not bring myself to say one or two months. For some reason, three months sounded less brutal.

Needless to say, we were all upset. But I knew from my experience that once Tracey and I had talked and shared why we loved one another, we were both relieved. I told Shelley that she was going to have to do something that would probably seem like the hardest thing she would ever have to do. "You need to go upstairs, hold your dad's hand, and tell him why you love him. Don't be afraid to cry, and don't be upset if he cries too. Tell him that you know he is dying, and that you will always love him. Let him talk with you so that he can share his feelings. You need to do this alone, without anyone else. For the past two years, your dad has protected us from his illness. He has given us the gift of wonderful memories. Now it is our turn to protect him."

I was amazed by Shelley's strength. Without hesitating, she walked upstairs and talked with Tracey for thirty minutes. Then, Connie spent time alone with Tracey. Even though they were divorced, they had shared ten years together. They had a wonderful daughter. They still loved and cared for each other. Everyone needed a chance to say good-bye.

Around 10 P.M., Connie and Shelley went home. Diane, Don, and I sat in our bedroom with Tracey. We watched TV and talked. By 11 P.M., Tracey was dozing off, and I began the ritual of saying good-night. Don and Diane went to bed. I turned off the lights and Tracey immediately became restless. He had taken a sedative but as time passed, he became more distressed. I had not slept in practically forty-eight hours and was exhausted. At midnight, I asked Diane to come upstairs and sit with Tracey so that I could get some sleep. Around 3 A.M., I went to the bathroom and peeked in our bedroom. Diane wasn't sitting in the chair, she was lying in our bed with her arm draped across Tracey. I laughed and later told Diane that I wouldn't let just any woman sleep with my husband. Unfortunately, Tracey was not sleeping soundly. Fifteen minutes later, Diane woke me up, "Tracey can't sleep and says he needs you." I sent Diane to bed and tried to make Tracey comfortable, but I was confused. The drugs did not seem to have any lasting effect. There had to be a reason for these panic attacks.

Friday was a blur of activity. Tracey's parents had spent the summer in Michigan, but they had left to visit friends in Pennsylvania before returning to their home in Florida. I had to tell them on the phone to come back to Detroit because Tracey was dying. Soon after, my cousin Barb arrived; she was shortly followed by Tracey's sister, Claudia, and his Aunt Dorothy. Barb served Tracey breakfast in bed while I talked with Claudia and Aunt Dorothy. I told them basically the same thing that I had told Shelley. As I finished talking with them, a representative from Hospice of Southeastern Michigan arrived. I was trying to function on about five hours of sleep over the past forty-eight hours, and I was having a hard time finding Tracey's insurance card, let alone making decisions. Thankfully, Barb took notes and asked the questions that needed to be asked. It was explained that a nurse, Stacey, and a social worker, Leah, would call and schedule a time to visit.

By 11 A.M., Stacey was sitting in our family room talking with me to identify our specific needs. She immediately recommended a sleeping pill to help Tracey rest. Next, a hospital bed and a portable toilet were ordered. Her van was a virtual medical supply storehouse—blue pads, a hospital gown, and bed sheets appeared. I was relieved, for I had access to someone who would give me practical advice. For the time being, Stacey would visit every couple of days, and arrangements were made to schedule a home care aide to help me for two hours, Monday through Friday. We were treated with compassion and respect. Stacey was genuinely interested in our family and made me feel like I was in control again. One of the most helpful things that I received was a booklet that described the stages of death, both physical and psychological. Knowing what to expect and what was considered normal was extremely helpful to me. This knowledge reduced my fears and allowed me to help family and friends. I encouraged everyone who visited to read it. Before she left, I told Stacey about Tracey's dream and asked if Hospice could help me contact Elton John so that Tracey could meet him at the concert in October. She said that she would talk with the Development Department and see what they could do. It was very evident that Tracey's strength was disappearing quickly. I was concerned about him even attending the concert in two weeks. Stacey told me, "Dying patients frequently save what little energy they have in order to see a dream come true. We will make sure that Tracey can get to the concert. We'll arrange for an ambulance, and we'll do our best to set up a meeting with Elton John."

At 4 P.M., I met the social worker, Leah. She outlined the basic services that could be provided and listened to my concerns. She explained that Hospice could also give assistance and counseling to other family members who needed it.

It had been a very long day. Claudia, Aunt Dorothy, and Barb were with us all day, so Tracey and I were both able to sleep. I was feeling much better. About 5 P.M., the night shift arrived. Tim and Rich, water-skiing friends, would spend the night. Sandy, Rich's wife, fixed lasagna for dinner. Stephanie, their seven year old daughter, and Tracey's little buddy, rounded out Friday night's visitors. After we ate, Tracey was more alert than I had seen him for a week. He wasn't talking a lot, but he watched and laughed at a Tim Allen comedy video. I had noticed that Tracey was fine as long as there was activity around him, and he had been able to sleep soundly during the day. I decided that I was going to take a different approach, and discussed my plan with Tim and Rich. They agreed to give it a try. We moved the La-Z-Boy chair and three lamps into the den. Instead of moving Tracey to the bed, he would sleep in the chair. The lights, the TV, and the radio would be on all night, and Rich and Tim would take turns staying with Tracey so that he would never be alone. We moved the couch next to the La-Z-Boy so that someone could hold his hand while he slept. At midnight, without saying a word, I disappeared and went to bed. If they needed me, they could wake me up. I dozed off, but was very restless. I got up to check on Tracey three or four times. It was very noisy in the den, and there was so much light that you almost needed sunglasses. Tracey and Tim were both sleeping. I couldn't believe it. For two weeks, all I wanted was for Tracey to sleep through the night. Now I was the one who could not sleep. I woke Tim and told him to go to bed. I'd sit with Tracey since I was awake anyway. For an hour, I watched him. By 4 A.M., I was pacing the hallway. I needed to talk with someone. I had read in the Hospice brochure that when a patient is getting ready to die, he becomes very peaceful. I was frantic, because I thought that Tracey was dying—right then and there. Tim sensed my movement in the hallway and asked me what was wrong. Rich heard the commotion and ran upstairs. I burst into tears and explained my fears between sobs. They put their arms around me for comfort, but our adrenaline had kicked in and there was no chance of any of us going back to sleep. We went to the den and watched TV. Meanwhile, Tracey never stirred. The next morning I was exhausted, but I was ecstatic. Through trial and error, I had identified the problem and discovered a solution. Just like a small child, the darkness and isolation of night scared Tracey. As long as the lights were on, there was background noise, and he was with someone he knew, he slept. I did not want to drug Tracey into submission. I wanted him to be aware of his surroundings and to feel our love. I had prayed for and received a miracle. Tracey never had a sleepless night again because our friends and family shared their love and strength with us. They gave us the priceless gift of unselfish courage.

By the time the sun rose, Tracey was famished and gobbled down breakfast. It was Saturday, and he had not showered since Monday morning. It took the strength of three people to help Tracey walk to the bathroom that was only about ten feet away.

By the time Tracey was clean and comfortably sitting in his chair again, we all were exhausted. At 11 A.M., the next shift arrived in the form of my cousins. Barb fixed lunch and started to clean my house. Jake and Barb's husband, Roger, were in charge of fixing the television in the den so that Tracey could watch cable TV. Scott, Brian, and Adam, my cousins' children, kept Uncle Tracey company. My family does not have a reputation for doing anything in a small way. Today was no exception. At noon, the portable toilet and the hospital bed were delivered. The bed was set up in the living room so that we would have more space and Tracey could see the lake. I decided that I would wait a couple of days before moving Tracey downstairs to the hospital bed. I needed to make sure that he continued to sleep through the night before I made any changes.

By 3 P.M., Tracey was exhausted from watching everybody. He didn't complain. He liked activity, but the pendulum had swung too far. I had gotten carried away, and Tracey let me know without hurting my feelings, that sometimes silence is golden.

Just as he was drifting off to sleep, his parents arrived. I knew that they wanted to spend time with him. I didn't want to hurt their feelings, but I told them that they would have to wait. Tracey needed to rest. They watched TV until he woke up. Then, one person at a time had a chance to talk with him. By Saturday evening, Tracey had said his good-byes to the most important people in his life, his family. From that point forward, he rarely had a conversation with anyone. It was very difficult for him to talk. His mask of silence allowed him to slowly withdraw from the world. This is not to say that I did not talk to Tracey. I'm sure sometimes he would have liked me to be quiet, but I decided he would let me know when enough was enough.

On Monday, an angel knocked on our door. Barbara, the Hospice home care aide, came to our rescue. I was unprepared to help a seriously ill person. Barbara taught me how to be a caregiver. She showed me how to change sheets, prevent bedsores, and give bed baths. She was a wonderful person with a gentle, calm demeanor. Without her guidance, I would have been lost, and Tracey would have suffered because of my inexperience. I was amazed by her capacity to relieve the discomfort of so many terminal patients. Through her competence and compassion, she eased my fear. She was an extraordinary person whose kindness I will never forget.

Doors are always open to share joy, but they are frequently locked when someone is facing death. I did not want Tracey to be isolated because of ignorance and fear. I wanted him to know that he was loved. The only way this could happen was if I encouraged and enabled others to visit. Visiting Tracey required unselfish courage. Everyone who walked through our door was afraid. They were fearful of the unknown. They were afraid of death. They didn't know what to say or how to act. Our first visitors stayed only fifteen minutes. It appeared that Tracey was tired, and his friends did not want to impose. Unknown to them, Tracey had instinctively closed his eyes to protect himself, for it hurt too much to see the pain in his friends' eyes. Immediately after his friends left, Tracey had an anxiety attack because he knew that he might never see them again. After this experience, everyone was welcome to visit by appointment, provided they agreed to one rule—they had to stay for at least two hours. This may have seemed unreasonable, but I was determined not to sedate Tracey in order to control his anxiety. In addition, I had to make sure that everyone had an opportunity to spend quality time with Tracey. Therefore, I had to limit the number of people who visited each day. Everyone was a little concerned, for what could they possibly do or say for two hours with someone who wouldn't talk or open his eyes? The answer was fairly simple. First, I suggested that people come in pairs. Second, I became Tracey's mouthpiece. Tracey and our company were always my priority. Everything else could wait.

I became a pseudo-counselor. I explained to each person, "It is very difficult for Tracey to speak. He may not say a word while you are here and he may not even open his eyes. I have talked with him and he has repeatedly told me that he wants company. If you try to put yourself in his place, imagine what it would be like to look into the tearful eyes of a friend. No matter how hard you try, you cannot hide The Look. Emotionally and physically, Tracey does not have the energy to deal with your sorrow, but he wants, he needs your love and friendship. Tell him, 'it's good to see you.' Talk about what you and your family are doing. Reminisce about the fun you have shared together. When it is time to leave, don't say 'good-bye.' Tracey does not do good-byes. If you need to say anything, tell him that you love him." Word spread among our friends, and during the next seven weeks, over one hundred people spent time with us, many coming more than once. Many times he was so quiet it appeared as if Tracey were sleeping. People were amazed when I would offer him something to eat or drink, and without saying a word or opening his eyes, he would open his mouth. I laughed at people's reactions and said, "Tracey is the 'Trickster.' He makes you think that he's not paying attention so that he can reel you in and find out your deepest secrets." Frequently, someone would be talking about sports or some current event, when out of nowhere Tracey would offer an opinion or make a wisecrack. He had always been able to get other people to laugh. Even as he faced death, his sense of humor never deserted him.

During September, October, and November, I frequently spent the entire day just sitting in the living room and talking with our friends. Sometimes we would watch a video. On other occasions, we would eat a meal together. If Tracey decided he had something to say, he would say it. Otherwise, he listened to his friends. Since he kept his eyes shut, he couldn't see their sorrow. He only heard the joy, the love, and the compassion in their voices. As each day passed, Tracey found an inner peace that was evident to every person who entered our home.

On the first of October, my sister, Carol, arrived from Arizona and stayed with us for ten days. Since she lived so far away, Tracey had never really had a chance to get to know her. I was thankful for her help and company. Our lives had been turned upside down, but we had finally settled into a comfortable routine. The center of my universe was Tracey, but I no longer felt that I was bearing this tragedy by myself. In addition to everyone who spent the night with Tracey, six women volunteered to spend one day a week with us. Beside keeping us company, they cleaned our house, went grocery shopping, and cooked meals. People were helping, not only because they loved Tracey, but because they also loved me. I knew that I was not alone.

In five days, we would be going to the Elton John concert. Hospice had not yet been successful in reaching Elton, but they were still trying. However, another problem surfaced when I realized that we could not go to the concert without help. We needed another ticket, but the Palace, where the concert was to occur, was sold out. Hospice was trying to get an additional ticket, but was not having any success. Remember RULE #1— ASK YOUR FRIENDS FOR HELP! I knew that my employer, Compuware Corporation, had a corporate suite available for the event, and I soon discovered that it had been reserved by the chairman, Peter Karmanos. I was not shy. I needed help. I talked to his secretary and explained my problem. Within an hour she called back and said, "Peter said that an executive from the Palace will call you this afternoon. He's sure that there will not be a problem getting another ticket." By 2 P.M., arrangements had been completed. Another roadblock had been removed, and we were on our way to the concert.

For two days, we listened to Elton John music non-stop. I tried to get Tracey to tell me his favorite song. He shook his head and said, "I don't have a favorite. I love all his music." Friday, October 6, 1995, finally arrived. I wanted to make sure that Tracey had a chance to rest, so no one was invited to visit. I helped Tracey choose his clothes, for he was still proud and wanted to look good. Almost everything was arranged. The concert would begin at 8 P.M., but in order to avoid crowds, we needed to be at the Palace by 6:15 P.M. My cousin, Jake, would leave from work and meet us at our seats. There was only one outstanding question—would we meet Elton John?

At 4 P.M., our phone rang. It was Katie, from the Hospice Development staff. She exclaimed, "Kathy! He said 'Yes!' Elton has agreed to meet Tracey before the concert!" We were both crying. I couldn't believe it. Tracey was going to meet Elton John. I decided to hold back the surprise until we were at the Palace, since I didn't want him to be disappointed if something happened.

We were transported by ambulance. Tammy, a Palace representative, met us at the door with a specially equipped wheelchair for Tracey. As we were escorted to our seats, Tammy mentioned, "I hope you don't mind, but we've changed your seats a little." I shrugged my shoulders. We didn't care where we sat; we were just glad to be there. Then I remembered Jake. How would he find us? Tammy said, "Don't worry. Security will find him and show him where you are seated."

As we moved along, I noticed that people were looking at us. They weren't staring. Instead, their eyes had an expression of excitement, for they knew that this was a special evening. Suddenly, I realized where we were going. Tracey had his eyes closed, but I leaned over and whispered in his ear, "Open your eyes honey. You've got to see where we are." We were standing next to the stage. In a few moments, we were joined by my cousin. He had been waiting for us at our original seats. Since the Palace was empty, he had seen us down on the floor. I was curious, "Where were our seats?" Jake pointed to a location I call heaven. We had been moved from the rafters to seats 001 and 002, the best in the house.

At 7 P.M., a security guard asked me to go backstage. The tour manager wanted to talk with me. As I waited, I held my breath. The tour manager introduced himself and said, "Elton wants to see you right here at 7:45 P.M." I could hardly wait to surprise Tracey. When I told him, he was speechless, but tears filled his eyes. Before we knew it, we were standing backstage. A curtain parted, and Elton appeared out of nowhere.

Even though he was a superstar, he was very gracious. You would never have guessed that he had a huge performance in a few minutes. We were the center of his universe. He kissed me on the cheek and then introduced himself to Tracey, "I'm so glad that you are able to come to my concert. It means a lot to me that you are here." He noticed that Tracey was holding his latest CD, *Made in England* and autographed it, "To Tracey with love, Elton." He talked with us for a few moments and asked Tracey if he had a favorite song. Tracey was overwhelmed, and could not talk. I shook my head. "Elton (we were on a first name basis; after all, he had kissed me), he doesn't have a favorite. He loves all your music." Elton smiled and remembered, "Oh, I have something for you," and handed me a large bag. Suddenly, Elton looked uncomfortable, until he extended his hand and introduced himself to Jake. "Excuse me for being so rude. I'm Elton John." He realized that there was a third person in our group and did not want to ignore anyone. As he turned to leave, he inquired, "Where are you sitting?" He seemed satisfied with my reply and waved good-bye.

The rest of the evening was a celebration filled with music, happiness, and love. We were about thirty feet from where Elton performed and played the piano. Everyone watched over us. Security prevented anyone from blocking our view and offered us beverages when Tracey looked tired. Complete strangers from the audience gave us roses and hugged us. They were aware, without anyone saying anything, that this was a special night.

During the performance, Elton did not say much at all. He let his music speak for him. At about 10 P.M., the band took a break and Elton sat down at the piano to play a solo. As he prepared to play a ballad, he looked in our direction. "Before this evening's performance, I had the privilege of meeting a remarkable couple backstage. I would like to dedicate this next song to Tracey and Kathy." His fingers began to move on the keyboard. The melody and lyrics enveloped us as he sang:

There's a calm surrender
To the rush of day
When the heat of a rolling world
Can be turned away.

An enchanted moment
And it sees me through
It's enough for this restless warrior
Just to be with you.

And can you feel the love tonight?
It is where we are
It's enough for this wide-eyed wanderer
That we got this far.
And can you feel the love tonight?
How it's laid to rest?
It's enough to make kings and vagabonds
Believe the very best.

There's a time for everyone
If they only learn
That the twisting kaleidoscope
Moves us all in turn
There's a rhyme and reason
To the wild outdoors
When the heart of this star-crossed voyager
Beats in time with yours

It's enough to make kings and vagabonds
Believe the very best.

Chapter Eighteen
Unselfish Courage

By the time we reached home, it was midnight. My sister Carol was waiting for us, and my cousin came back to our house to help. As Jake came into the living room, he wanted to know, "Kathy, what's in the bag?" I had been so caught up in the excitement of the evening that I had totally forgotten about the bag Elton had given to us. It took a moment to find. As I emptied its contents, we were thrilled. There was a concert program, a baseball cap with "ELTON JOHN" emblazoned across the brim, and five different tour T-shirts. We were all on a natural high. As Tracey drifted off to sleep, I tried to tell Carol about our celebration. If I had not experienced the evening myself, I would have thought it had been a dream, but this dream had more than come true.

We were expecting company the next day. As Tracey was eating breakfast, he asked, "Can I tell people about Elton John?" I told him, "That's a great idea." Tracey had a knack for telling stories, and he never told a story the same way twice. The adventures always got bigger and better. Unfortunately, Tracey couldn't tell anyone about the Elton John concert. He couldn't tell stories anymore; brain cancer wouldn't let him. Instead, I became Tracey, and told visitor after visitor about our wonderful anniversary night. Even though Tracey did not say a word or open his eyes, his face could not hide the emotions he held deep inside. Exaggeration wasn't necessary. The real story was too wonderful, and it was retold by many people who shared it with their friends.

Since Tracey's dream had been fulfilled, I was afraid that he would die within two weeks. His anxiety attacks completely disappeared—except when I left the house to run an errand. I decided that unless it was absolutely necessary, I would not go anywhere. Over a seven week period, I left the house only six times for about an hour each time. I did not feel confined or isolated because everyone was coming to our house. Friends asked, "Doesn't all this company drive you crazy." But I thought it was wonderful to be surrounded by so much concern and love. Many people encouraged me to go to the movies, or out to dinner, but I refused. I couldn't leave Tracey. I could not save his life, but I could make sure that he was not afraid as long as he lived.

The few instances I did go out involved making funeral arrangements. I am a planner and only feel comfortable if I am organized. Tracey had told me where he wanted to be buried, but I needed to choose a funeral home and select a casket. Fortunately, the director of the funeral home was very helpful and sympathetic. He made the whole process bearable. There were details that needed to be handled and I had time and friends who were willing to help. Tracey wanted people to remember him as he was in life—full of energy. After sorting through all our photo albums, I asked my friend Barb to make a collage. In addition, one photo was enlarged into a portrait. I knew that I wanted a special eulogy and asked Kay, a writer, to help me. I called my brother Denis, a talented musician, and asked for suggestions regarding music. I wanted to have a reception, and Marge offered to find some possible locations. The primary problem was that we did not belong to a church. However, over the past two years, the pastors of Metropolitan United Methodist Church, Dr. William Quick and Dr. J. D. Landis, had become our friends. They had visited Tracey in the hospital and at our home. They had wanted and encouraged us to join their congregation. Even though we didn't join, they continued to offer their help and prayers. At first, I was thankful, because their visits had a calming effect on Tracey, and I appreciated their friendship. Gradually, J. D. Landis's quiet, warm manner overcame my resistance. He slowly drew me into a circle of prayer and peace. As soon as I asked him, J. D. agreed to preside at the funeral service.

The major arrangements were made, and I could concentrate on Tracey. I was taking care of his basic needs. He was not physically suffering, and there was no pain or discomfort. He could no longer feed himself, but still he had a hearty appetite. Friends brought his favorite foods. Simple chewing took a lot of energy, and meals often lasted an hour or more.

I was constantly aware of any changes in Tracey's moods and appearance. Early in our marriage, Tracey had affectionately nicknamed me "the Inspector," because I was always examining him. At first, he thought that I was looking for flaws, but after awhile he realized that I was just curious. I couldn't help myself. Now, I was on constant alert. I tried to put myself in his shoes and anticipate what he might want or need. In order to alleviate possible boredom, I played music and read to him. We told each other that we loved one another, but I realized one day that I had become his caregiver. The passion and playfulness, always a part of our relationship as husband and wife, were missing. This was not surprising since Tracey was so ill. He didn't move without assistance and rarely talked or opened his eyes—even with me. I decided that we needed a date, a night alone together. One Saturday evening, I played soft music and served a romantic dinner by candlelight. The whole evening, Tracey never opened his eyes or spoke a word. After dessert, there was still no reaction. Finally, I leaned over and gave Tracey a passionate kiss, and he responded by returning my kiss. I knew then that even though Tracey did not seem to be aware, the man I loved was alive and still needed the passion that we shared. On another occasion, I had given Tracey some chocolate pudding. Because I had not done a very neat job of feeding him, his lips were smeared with chocolate. I always had a towel handy, but this day I startled him by licking the pudding off his face. It had been weeks since Tracey had laughed. This day, he not only laughed, but he smiled too.

Near the end of October, Tracey and I had two brief conversations. The first occurred as he had his last anxiety attack. I was totally perplexed. It was the middle of the afternoon, and we were alone. I couldn't imagine what had caused him to become upset. I tried to reassure him and asked him what was wrong. He opened his eyes and after a moment said, "I'm ruining your life." He was worried about me. The look in his eyes told me he wanted to say more but couldn't. I kissed him tenderly on the forehead and whispered, "Tracey, I know you feel like I am the only one who is giving, but you are wrong. You don't realize what you have given me. Before I met you, I thought I would never be able to love and trust anyone again. You taught me how to love and trust when I didn't think it was possible. For the past two years, you have protected me from your illness so that I will only remember how wonderful our life has been together. You have given me more than I ever expected." Tears were flowing down my face. Tracey closed his eyes. He was at peace as he repeated three words, "Protect . . . trust . . . love."

A few days later, we were alone again. In a very tired voice, Tracey told me, "Kathy, I don't want to fight any more." I had been warned that this might happen. Tracey was asking for my permission to die. My eyes said, "I don't want you to die. Please don't leave me." But my voice said, "Honey, you've been fighting for a long time. You don't need to fight any more." My heart was not ready to let go, but I was able to say the words I thought he needed to hear.

One day when Shelley came to visit, I warned her that Tracey might also ask for her permission to die. She needed to be prepared. Four days a week, she came to spend time with her father. I was worried about her because she was continuing with her college courses and working part-time. She was burning the candle at both ends. I told her that I was concerned, and didn't want her to get sick. If she felt overwhelmed, she should consider reducing her hours at work or dropping some of her classes. Her health was the most important thing. She was adamant and wanted to continue school and work. If it got to be too much, she would let her mom and me know. I was amazed by her determination. For being only twenty-one years old, Shelley was remarkably courageous and strong.

Two weeks passed and my birthday, November 1, was quickly approaching. I was afraid that Tracey would die on my birthday, but he continued to survive. Where was he getting this strength? On Sunday, November 5, both of our families visited— twenty-five people in one day. It was an all-time record. Everybody wanted to celebrate my birthday as well as Tracey's, which was November 21. It was a very busy day filled with the people who loved us the most.

Another important family event was drawing near. Tracey's brother, Michael, was getting married on November 17. The wedding had been planned for over a year, and I knew the bride and groom were apprehensive. What would happen if Tracey died? I knew that Tracey did not want his illness to interfere. Since there was no way to predict how long Tracey would live, I told everyone that if Tracey died the week of Michael and Sue's wedding, I would postpone the funeral until after the ceremony. Everyone was relieved that a decision had been made.

On Monday, November 6, Tracey was lethargic and was having trouble swallowing. I thought he was tired from Sunday's activity. However, by Tuesday, he was only eating very soft foods and could no longer take fluids with a straw. I had to use an eyedropper to give him juice and water. On Thursday, swallowing anything was impossible. Kirk, a boyhood friend of Tracey's, came to visit, but for the first time, no one could think of anything to say. The atmosphere was very depressing. I decided we needed to do something, and asked Kirk to help me get our Christmas tree out of the attic. Tracey's dad helped string the lights, and Shelley began decorating the tree. As we hung each ornament, we laughed and shared memories of previous holidays. As Christmas carols played on the stereo, everyone's spirits were lifted. That evening, I told Tracey that I wanted to open a present that had been placed on our fireplace five weeks ago. I had avoided opening it, but I couldn't wait any longer. The time was right. I slowly removed the gold ribbon and the embroidered wrapping paper. The lettering on the outside of the box read "Final Edition." It was the Waterford crystal ornament, Twelve Drummers Drumming, that completed my "Twelve Days of Christmas" collection. I would always treasure this gift.

On Friday morning, Stacey, the Hospice nurse, came to check Tracey's vital signs. When the examination was complete, we walked into the kitchen to talk. Stacey was very gentle, but she knew that I needed to know what to expect. "Since Tracey has stopped eating and is unable to swallow, I know that he is entering the final stages. His heart is still very strong and his blood pressure has not dropped significantly. Based on my experience, it will probably be a few days before he dies. I will come back on Monday, but if you need help or have questions, don't hesitate to call the Hospice phone number." She hugged me good-bye, and I returned to the living room and held my best friend's hand.

As the day passed, I related to our family what Stacey had said. They could see that Tracey was not suffering, but it seemed harsh not to provide fluids with an IV. I explained that his body was shutting down, and if we tried to provide nourishment, he would become uncomfortable. His body would not know how to handle any fluids which were not needed or expected. Friday night, I tried to give Tracey some water with an eye dropper. The only thing I accomplished was making him cough for thirty minutes. It was very difficult to do nothing. At 11 P.M., I kissed Tracey good-night and walked upstairs to the bedroom. Our friend, Mark, spent the night holding Tracey's hand. Early the next morning, it poured rain, changed to sleet, and then began to snow. Mark was going hunting up North and needed to leave at 7 A.M. I fixed a pot of coffee as he went out to warm up his car. I went downstairs to the family room to turn on the stereo. When Mark came back inside, he looked at my face and knew that something was wrong. I was standing at the top of the stairway and began to cry, "The basement flooded again. The sump pump didn't kick on." This was more than I could handle, and by this time we were standing at the foot of Tracey's bed. Mark put his arms around me and I sobbed into his shoulder, "Tracey doesn't want to be like this. I wish that he would die." I was finally ready to let Tracey go. He had my permission to die.

Mark fixed the pump, by adjusting a lever, and the water quickly drained. We moved everything off the floor and wiped up the standing water with towels. It appeared that we had discovered the problem before the carpet had been soaked. Finally, Mark left at 10 A.M. I started calling everyone who was scheduled to visit to tell them not to come. The house was a disaster. For the first time in seven weeks, I did not want company. The roads were treacherous; I tried to reach Shelley, but she was already on her way. I couldn't believe the unseasonable weather. It was too soon to be snowing. It was only November 11. Shelley stayed for two hours. When she left, I sat by Tracey's side for the rest of the day. I talked to him for hours. It was a one-sided conversation, but I knew that he could still hear me. I reminisced about how we met and fell in love. I recalled special memories that we alone shared, and played all of his favorite music. When I couldn't think of anything more to say, I decided that I would read his eulogy aloud. I had been surprised that it had not been difficult to write. More than anything, I wanted his funeral to be a celebration of his life. His eulogy needed to reflect his strength and courage. I wanted people to nod and say, "That was the Tracey I knew and loved." The day passed quickly and the shadows of evening descended. I opened the drapes and looked out on the silent night. An inch of snow had accumulated, and I turned on the Christmas tree lights. It was very peaceful.

At 8 P.M., my cousin, Jenny, and her husband, Pete, arrived. They were Tracey's roommates for the night. They were going to retire in seven months, and we talked about their plans to sail around the world. About 10:30 P.M., I mentioned that I was concerned about Tracey, and thought that I would sleep in the chair next to him. Jenny tried to convince me that if anything happened she would wake me, but I was not persuaded. His breathing was labored. Was this what they called the death rattle? Jenny didn't think so. Tracey seemed very calm. Nothing was wrong. But as I was getting out the bed linens for us, there was a very strong aroma around Tracey. It was very noticeable but not anything I could identify. It was not fragrant or foul. It was just different. The aroma did not permeate the room. You had to be within two feet of Tracey to smell it. I decided this had to be a result of Tracey's not eating for three days. At 11 P.M., I remembered that Tracey needed to take his seizure pill. I turned on the lights so that I could see. After I had administered his medication, I noticed a major change. Tracey's face had lost its fullness and pink coloring. His cheeks looked hollow. I looked at Jenny and said, "I think Tracey is dying." She did not agree, "No, he's fine." I moved to the other side of the bed and pushed the chair away so that I was only two inches away from his face. Tracey took a deep breath and paused. I repeated, "I think he's dying." Again, Jenny disagreed, "No, he's just got some mucous in his throat." Tracey took another deep breath and paused. I was not saying anything and Jenny said, "Kathy, talk to Tracey." I shook my head no. There was nothing left for me to tell him. I put my arms around my husband, and began to pray aloud:

Our Father, Who art in heaven, hallowed be Thy name; Thy kingdom come; Thy will be done on earth as it is in heaven. Give us this day our daily bread; and forgive us our trespasses, as we forgive those who trespass against us; and lead us not into temptation, but deliver us from evil. For Thine is the kingdom, the power, and the glory, now and forever. Amen.

Hail, Mary, full of grace; the Lord is with thee; blessed art thou among women, and blessed is the fruit of thy womb, Jesus. Holy Mary, Mother of God, pray for us sinners, now and at the hour of our death. Amen.

Glory be to the Father, and to the Son, and to the Holy Spirit. As it was in the beginning, is now, and ever shall be, world without end.

As I said the final amen, Tracey took his last breath and died in my arms. The time was 11:11 P.M. on November 11. I began to cry and laid my head on Tracey's chest. His strong heart was no longer beating. I raised myself and noticed that there was a haze across Tracey's cheekbones. Thinking that my vision was blurred, I rubbed my eyes. I squinted, moved closer, and tried to figure out what I was seeing. It was as if I was looking through heavy plastic. This haze, or glow, lasted only for a few moments, and when it vanished, the strange aroma I had noticed around Tracey disappeared too.

I wanted to remember every detail. It was like I became a detached observer and began to notice other physical changes in Tracey. His nails turned purple and then suddenly were white; his skin became mottled where blood began to settle; his body absorbed my body heat wherever I touched him.

I was not frightened. The closest I can come to describing my feelings is that my whole body and soul were grieving. I knew that I would need to let Tracey go, but I was not going to be rushed. For about twenty minutes, I simply laid my upper body across Tracey's and mourned my loss.

I had talked with our family about Tracey's death and knew their wishes. I rose and called Shelley. She wanted to see her father before his body was moved from our home. As we waited for her to arrive, Jenny, Pete, and I bathed Tracey for the last time and changed the linen. I wanted Shelley to sense the peace that had come to Tracey with death. When she arrived, we hugged and I briefly explained how and when he had died. Together, we held Tracey. After a few minutes, I left the room. Shelley needed to grieve alone. When she was finished saying good-bye and was sure that I would not be alone, Shelley left. I returned and kept a vigil at Tracey's side.

I was on my own timetable. There was no hurry. Since I had been briefed beforehand, nothing unexpected happened. At about midnight, I called Hospice and was told that someone would come immediately. Legally, the police also needed to document Tracey's death. I had asked a friend, Ron, who was a policeman, if he would help me when Tracey died. I didn't want to deal with strangers and have to answer questions. Even though it was very difficult for him, Ron, like so many others, wanted to help us any way he could. Mercifully, when the police came, Ron handled all the details and I did not need to be involved. A Hospice nurse arrived, and at 12:40 A.M., November 12, 1995, Tracey was pronounced dead.

The sorrow in our home was like a heavy fog. It permeated everyone and everything. The Hospice nurse asked permission to call the funeral home. I nodded, knowing that Tracey would soon be leaving our home for the last time. At about 2:30 A.M., there was a knock at the door. Two men quietly expressed their condolences and waited for me to give them directions. I had always worried about this moment, for I thought that I wouldn't be able to stay in the room when Tracey's body was removed. However, the opposite occurred. I couldn't leave. I stood at the end of the hospital bed with my arms folded across my chest. I was not finished protecting Tracey. He had been hurt many times, and I was going to make sure that he was carefully transferred from the bed to the gurney. If they were not gentle, I would not allow them to touch Tracey. My misgivings were unfounded, because they cautiously wrapped him in a white sheet and lifted him onto the cart. I remember thinking, "Tracey looks so sweet. He looks like a baby wrapped in swaddling clothes." I gently cradled Tracey's face in my hands and lightly kissed him on the forehead. Tracey's body left our home, but his spirit of love remained. My greatest fear did not come to pass; I did not feel that I was alone.

Chapter Ninteen

When We Open Our Hearts

For so long, all my attention had been focused on Tracey and the details surrounding his death. I was in my own private world and had been oblivious to everyone around me. As I closed the sliding glass door, a feeling of relief came over me. Tracey's suffering was over. But when I turned and saw Jenny, Pete, and Ron standing across the room, I experienced The Look for the first time. The sympathy and grief in their eyes and faces pierced my heart. I thought to myself, "No wonder Tracey closed his eyes." Their sadness overwhelmed me. Unlike Tracey, I was able to hug them and tell them, "It's okay." I was sad, but I was not devastated. After we talked for a few minutes, I kissed them and thanked them for their help. We were all emotionally and physically exhausted. It was 3 A.M. We said good-night, and I went to bed. Within seconds, I slept.

I awoke at 5 A.M.; I was not looking forward to what I had to do. I needed to tell Tracey's family that he had died. Tracey's folks were staying with his sister, Claudia, and I wanted to break the news in person. They were early risers, so I planned to go to Claudia's house by 7:30 A.M.

As I was getting ready, I replayed the details of Tracey's death in my mind. Gradually, I began to recall unusual events that had occurred during the past three days. Suddenly, everything that I had perceived made sense. Some people may feel that what I am going to relate is how I am handling my grief, that my imagination is working overtime, or that I have gone off the deep end. However, I am confident that what I saw and heard was real.

On Thursday, November 9, I was alone with Tracey for part of the day. As I was quietly sitting next to him, I heard unexplained noises under his bed. I noticed the sounds but ignored them. Later, I heard them again and even looked under the bed. Finding nothing, I decided I was hearing things and turned on the stereo.

That evening, I was in my bedroom getting ready to go to bed. The door was ajar and in my peripheral vision, I saw a shadow move in the hallway. I remember turning my head and thinking, "What was that?" Since Tracey and Rich were both downstairs in the living room, I knew there was nothing there.

At about 3 A.M. the following night, I was awakened from a deep sleep by a 'thunk' on my bedroom door. I got out of bed and went into the hallway, but no one was there. I looked down the stairway and saw that both Mark and Tracey were in the living room and fast asleep. Again, I dismissed what had happened, thinking I must have been dreaming.

Sunday morning, Jenny mentioned that she had briefly smelled an unusual odor around Tracey. As I thought about these events in conjunction with the aroma and haze that I had encountered on Saturday night, I realized that I had seen Tracey's spirit leave his body. I am convinced that the noises and shadow were a spiritual being who was trying to let me know that Tracey would soon die. I feel that God knew I would ignore the haze, just like I ignored the other signs in our home. In order to get my attention, He gave me concrete evidence that what I saw and heard was real. The proof was that both Jenny and I smelled this strange aroma which disappeared with Tracey's spirit. No one else saw the haze. If I had not been so sensitive to the physical changes in Tracey, I probably would have missed it too.

As I continued to think about Tracey's death, I realized that there were other coincidences. Over the last seven weeks, every day had seen a constant stream of visitors. In retrospect, I realized that neither Shelley nor I had much of an opportunity to be alone with Tracey. If our lower level had not flooded, and had there not been a snowstorm, we would have had company all day. Tracey's favorite season was winter. He loved snow. Each year he could hardly wait to set up the Christmas tree. On Saturday, for some reason, I played all of the music which had been a source of inspiration and encouragement for Tracey. On the last day of his life, Tracey had everything that he loved—music, snow, Christmas, and his family.

Then, the depth of Tracey's love hit me like a ton of bricks. Tracey had wanted to die long before he did. He told me so. However, he could not let go of his earthly body until he knew I would be all right. On Saturday morning, he had heard me say, "I wish that Tracey would die," but he did not want me to be alone when he died. So he waited. He knew that when I gave him his night medication, someone would be with me. Eleven minutes after I gave him his seizure pill, he took his last breath. For two years, Tracey had protected me from his illness. In spite of multiple surgeries, radiation, chemotherapy, and paralysis, he enthusiastically greeted every day. He appreciated everything that people did for him, but expected nothing. And now, at the time of his death, he thought only of protecting me. I was overwhelmed.

For the first time in my life, I had an urgent need to go to church. I had been given the gift of unconditional love, and I had to give thanks to God in His house. Sunday service at Metropolitan United Methodist Church was not until 11 A.M. This gave me the time I needed to spend with Tracey's family. Even though they had long known that Tracey could die at anytime, it did not lessen their grief. We hugged one another, and were thankful that Tracey was not suffering anymore. After awhile, I excused myself. This was going to be a very busy day.

I attended church and then met with J.D. Landis after the service. I had to share with him what had happened. He listened intently and accepted my story without question. He was amazed that I had come to church so soon after Tracey's death. My response was, "After what has happened, how can I be anywhere else?"

When I came home, I began to call family and friends to let them know that Tracey passed away. I knew that everyone would want to know the details of Tracey's death, but I did not have time to tell each person individually. To solve my dilemma, I invited people to come over Sunday night. By 8:30 P.M., there were over twenty people sitting in our living room. All of these friends had helped care for Tracey, and they were all mourning. Any one of them could have been with him when he died. Until tonight, most of these people had never met one another. Their common bond was their love for Tracey and me. I asked everyone to introduce themselves and to explain how they knew

Tracey. This gave everyone a chance to get to know something about Tracey they may have not known. It also allowed everyone to share their grief. An hour later, I began to talk. I wanted to make sure that each person realized what they had done for our family. "It took real courage for you to help Tracey. Without you, our lives would have been hell. The love that Tracey needed was more than one person could give. Many of you loved Tracey at night so that I could love him during the day. Your unconditional love saved his spirit and allowed him to die in peace. Without your help, I would have been an empty shell and would have been devastated by his death. You may not realize it, but you saved my life, too. I will always love you."

I then told them how Tracey had died. When I finished, each person had been able to experience Tracey's death. It was as if the clock had been turned back and it was Saturday, November 11, at 11:11 P.M. There were no questions, only silence. No one wanted to break the spell. No one was ashamed of the tears in their eyes. They knew that Tracey was safe.

At midnight, I finally had to push everyone out the door. It had been a wonderful evening, but I needed sleep. My friend Diane would not leave, and said she was going to spend the night. I was too tired to argue and set my alarm for 6:20 A.M., because Diane needed to go to work. As soon as my head hit the pillow, I was sound asleep. By 5 A.M., I was wide awake. It was too early to get up, so I decided to just lie in bed. I missed Tracey and needed his touch. I thought about what had happened over the past three days. I was convinced that Tracey was still with me and asked him, "Put your arms around me so that I can feel you. I know that you can embrace me." I closed my eyes and waited. Nothing happened, and I was disappointed. I stayed in bed, and when the radio came on at 6:20, the very first word of my favorite song was playing. Tracey was the only person who knew that this was my favorite song. I can't describe the joy I felt as I listened to the lyrics of "Fields of Gold."

> You'll remember me
> When the West wind moves
> Upon the fields of barley
> You'll forget the sun in its jealous sky
> As we walk in fields of gold
>
> So she took her love
> For to gaze awhile

Upon the fields of barley
In his arms she fell
As her hair came down
Among the fields of gold

Will you stay with me
Will you be my love
Among the fields of barley
You'll forget the sun in its jealous sky
As we lie in fields of gold

See the West wind move
Like a lover's soul
Upon the fields of barley
Feel her body rise
When you kiss her mouth
Among the fields of gold

I never made promises lightly
And there have been some that I've broken
But I swear in the days still left
We'll walk in fields of gold
We walk in fields of gold

Many years have passed
Since those summer days
Among the fields of barley
See the children run
As the sun goes down
Among the fields of gold.

You'll remember me
When the West wind moves
Upon the fields of barley
You can tell the sun in the jealous sky
That we walked in fields of gold
That we walked in fields of gold
That we walked in fields of gold.

At the conclusion of the song, I leapt out of bed. I had to tell
Diane what had just happened. Suddenly, for a reason I can't
explain, I laid back down. The next tune began. I immediately

recognized the upbeat melody, but until now I had never paid any attention to the lyrics. As I closed my eyes, I listened to Billy Joel sing, "The Longest Time."©

Oh, oh, oh
For the longest time
Oh, oh, oh
For the longest time

If you said good-bye to me tonight
There would still be music left to write
What else could I do
I'm so inspired by you
That hasn't happened for the longest time

Once I thought my innocence was gone
Now I know that happiness goes on
That's where you found me
When you put your arms around me
I haven't been there for the longest time

Oh, oh, oh
For the longest time
Oh, oh, oh
For the longest time

I'm that voice you're hearing in the hall
And the greatest miracle of all
Is how I need you
And how you needed me too
That hasn't happened for the longest time

Maybe this won't last very long
But you feel so right
And I could be wrong
Maybe I've been hoping too hard
But I've gone this far
And it's more than I hoped for

Who knows how much further we'll go on
Maybe I'll be sorry when you're gone
I'll take my chances
I forgot how nice romance is

I haven't been there for the longest time
I had second thoughts at the start
I said to myself
Hold on to your heart
Now I know the woman that you are
You're wonderful so far
And it's more than I hoped for

I don't care what consequence it brings
I have been a fool for lesser things
I want you so bad
I think you ought to know that
I intend to hold you for
The longest time.

At that moment, my life changed. If there had ever been any doubt, there was no longer. I knew that Tracey's spirit was still with me, and he was watching over me. For the longest time, brain cancer had prevented Tracey from telling me how much he loved me. It must have broken his heart to listen to me as I shared the reasons why I loved him, because he could not tell me how precious I was to him. It was not a coincidence that I heard these two songs. "Fields of Gold" was to get my attention. Tracey couldn't physically embrace me, but he held me through the music we both loved. He was again able to reach out and tell me that he needed me too.

The next week flew by, for our family would celebrate Michael and Sue's marriage in six days. Since I wanted to limit the impact of Tracey's death on their celebration, I delayed the funeral until November 21, Tracey's forty-sixth birthday. In a way, postponing the funeral was a blessing. The delay gave us time to notify all of our friends and family. Denise, Tracey's cousin, helped me organize everything and finalize the details. Before I knew it, the day that I would have to publicly say my last good-bye to Tracey arrived. Many times over the previous two years, I had said to myself, "How can I do this?" Somehow, somewhere I found the inner strength to deal with Tracey's illness, to tell Tracey he was dying, and to hold Tracey as he died. But surely, his funeral would be the worst day of my life. As I walked down the aisle of the church, I could not look to the left or right. My eyes were focused on the front of the church where Tracey's portrait was placed next to his casket. I sat in the front pew and waited.

J.D. Landis officiated. I was consoled by the prayers and scripture that he selected, but I was comforted most by his sermon. It was a strong message about determination, hope, and God's love. Music was blended into the ceremony by my brother, Denis, and my friend, Joyce. They sang Tracey's favorite songs. The eulogy was planned for the middle of the service. It had to be given by someone who knew and loved Tracey, and I smiled as Matt began:

Tracey Dennis Tuson was born November 21, 1949. He will always live in our memories whether these moments were shared as a husband, a father, a family member, or a friend.

Many of our memories of Tracey will make us laugh. Tracey loved to tell stories, some might call them tall tales. In any case, one of his favorites was a story about identical twins. One was an optimist. "Everything is coming up roses," he would say. The other was a sad and hopeless pessimist. He thought that Murphy, as in Murphy's Law, was an optimist. The worried parents of the boys brought them to the local psychologist. He suggested to the parents a plan to balance the twins' personalities. "On their next birthday, put them in separate rooms to open gifts. Give the pessimist the best toys you can afford and give the optimist a box of manure." The parents followed these instructions and carefully observed the results. When they peeked in on the pessimist they heard him complaining, "I don't like the color of this computer . . . I bet this Game Boy will break . . . I don't like this game . . . " Tiptoeing across the hall, the parents peeked in and saw their little optimist gleefully throwing the manure up in the air. He was laughing and told his parents, "You can't fool me! Where there's this much manure, there's gotta be a pony!"[1]

Tracey was just like this little optimist, except for one thing. He would have convinced his friends to join him in that pile of manure. His enthusiasm for all his interests—music, snow skiing, golf, water-skiing and nature—was contagious. He always wanted others to join in the fun. He once said that he felt that his urgency to play was a result of his childhood recovery from polio. At the age of five, he spent six months in an iron lung. For

---

[1] Author Unknown. The Optimist. *More Sower's Seeds*, Brian Cavanaugh.

two more years, he watched other children run and play before he was able to join them. As he grew, he not only tried to make up for lost time, but he also made sure that everyone he touched would share his excitement.

Competition became his middle name. He wanted to be the best at work as well as at play. If you ever visited Tracey at Sears, he was always glad to talk with you, unless of course, he sensed a sale. In mid-sentence, he would disappear and dash across the sales floor in hot pursuit of a potential customer. For twenty years, he convinced people over and over again that "You get more with a Kenmore."

Tracey's competitive spirit came alive with all sports. A friend once said, "Tracey is the best all-around athlete I've ever known." He relished beating his friends at golf and ski racing but was the first to congratulate you if you won.

The drive to win helped Tracey to battle his toughest foe for more than two years. Anyone who spent any time with Tracey during this period was amazed by his strength. His enthusiasm for life enabled him to make plans and genuinely anticipate what tomorrow held in store. Even the knowledge that he was dying did not stop him from looking forward to his dreams that would still come true. Kathy has asked me to share how Tracey faced his own mortality with unselfish courage.

In early September of this year, Tracey was having more and more trouble walking. As the day for his next CAT scan approached, he began to have anxiety attacks which were as horrible as any physical pain. His physicians admitted him to the hospital, performed tests and prescribed medication to provide relief. However, his nights remained sleepless. The tests showed that two brain tumors had reappeared. During the day Tracey slept because he was exhausted, and so the doctors were unable to tell him the disappointing results. The night before he was discharged, Tracey was so agitated that Kathy pushed him around the hospital in his wheelchair for two hours. Finally, Tracey settled down and in a peaceful moment, looking out on the city lights, Kathy told Tracey what he already knew in his heart. He simply whispered, "Oh, no!" He paused for just a moment and was immediately concerned about his daughter, Shelley, and his family. How could they bear the devastating news?

Kathy and Tracey talked about their life together and how lucky they were to have loved and been loved. A calmness settled over Tracey and he was able to sleep peacefully for the first time in weeks. Later in the morning, Tracey was quietly eating breakfast when he looked up and said, "You know I still have a dream that will come true." Kathy asked him what he meant. He smiled and said, "I've always wanted to see Elton John perform live and we have tickets for his concert." Even though he had just been told he was dying, his optimistic outlook enabled him to throw that box of manure up in the air and find that pony.

Through the help of many people, Tracey was able not only to enjoy the concert but also to meet Elton backstage and have front row seats for the performance. It was a celebration filled with music, happiness, and love. This kind of memory sustains us and reminds us that when we open our hearts to others we are never alone.

Tracey loved his family and friends with his whole heart and soul. Wonderful memories are his gift to us. In spite of the multiple surgeries, radiation, chemotherapy, and paralysis, he never complained or felt sorry for himself. He greeted every day with enthusiasm and a lust for life. We will remember how he made us laugh. We won't forget his competitive spirit and his unselfish courage. But most of all, we will remember that he loved us.

Tracey Dennis Tuson was born November 21, 1949. I loved Tracey. We will all miss him.

After the eulogy, there was one more message. I wanted to thank everyone who had the courage to love and to help Tracey and me. My friend, Sue, read a letter that I wrote:

Dearest Family and Friends,

As Tracey approached the end of his life, he reflected on how lucky he was and was able to say good-bye to his family and many of his friends. When he knew his body was failing, he became anxious and frightened, especially as evening approached. He needed to be protected. His friends and family rescued his spirit. You surrounded us with your love and shared your strength. Darkness became the light of day and fear was replaced by a sense of peace.

Tracey and I feel that this short verse describes the love and friendship that you so unselfishly gave.

> Somewhere in the darkest night
> There always shines
> A little light

This light
Up in the heavens
Shines
To help our God watch over us
When small children are born
The light
Their soul does adorn
So when our only human eyes
Look up into the lightless skies
We must know
Even though we cannot see
This light burns far into the night
To help our God watch over us

Thank you for guiding Tracey past the darkness of loneliness and despair. You gave him the ray of light that calmed his spirit and allowed him to meet his God in peace.

Tracey was my heart and soul

He was my North, my South, my East, and West,
My working week and my Sunday rest,
My noon, my midnight, my talk, my song;
I thought that love would last for ever: . . .

And it has.

Tracey and I Love You All.

At the end of the service, everyone came to the front of the church and passed by the casket. Until this point, I had not been aware that over two hundred and fifty people had come. As the procession of friends passed by, I was overcome with happiness and joy. I realized that these people had not only come to pay their last respects to Tracey, but they had also come because they loved me. I thought that Tracey's funeral would be the worst day of my life, but in fact, it felt like one of the best. I knew that Tracey's spirit was still with me, and I knew that I was loved. I was not alone. I suddenly realized the true meaning of the unselfish courage I had witnessed many times over the past two years. Unselfish courage is the gift of unconditional love that we give and receive when we open our hearts to others.

Postscript

A week following the funeral, I met my in-laws for lunch. George, my father-in-law, seemed a little nervous. I couldn't imagine what was bothering him. I hoped that I hadn't offended him. He hesitated for a moment and then began, "I want to talk to you about something that was said in the eulogy. You know, the part where Matt talked about Tracey having polio." I nodded my head and he continued, "Well, Tracey had polio all right, but he was never in an iron lung and was only in the hospital for about three weeks. Where did you ever hear that Tracey spent six months in an iron lung?"

It took about five seconds for me to absorb this new information, and suddenly I burst out laughing and shook my head. I couldn't believe that I had swallowed Tracey's biggest tall tale hook, line, and sinker. He only mentioned his bout with polio a couple of times. It wasn't something he normally discussed. For over thirteen years, I had listened to him exaggerate his adventures and always rolled my eyes when he embellished the truth. But I always believed his polio story.

I could just imagine that Tracey was laughing, too. Not only did he fool me, but I unwittingly convinced his largest audience, the people who attended his funeral, that this gross exaggeration was the truth. Friends had casually mentioned, "I didn't know that Tracey had polio as a child." Family members were confused, because they couldn't remember visiting Tracey in the hospital when he was in an iron lung. They whispered among themselves, "I'm sure that I would have remembered." Even Tracey's neurosurgeon and nurse, who attended the funeral, never questioned this implausible declaration. They simply looked at one another and said, "Did you know that?" But the best part of this joke was that I had convinced the pastor, J.D. Landis, that the iron lung episode was true. Needless to say, he was a little embarrassed. When I told him, he had a chagrined look and said, "Oh Kathy! I try so hard to make sure that everything that I say is true. I even asked you about it twice because it just didn't ring true." I laughed, "I swear that I thought it was true too. What's really hilarious is not only that I mentioned it in the eulogy, but you talked at length in the sermon about Tracey's bravery in the face of such overwhelming odds. No one would ever question your integrity. From what I can gather, I may be the only person whom Tracey told about the iron lung."

Thinking back to the day Tracey died, I recalled reading his eulogy to him. Although he didn't say a word, I know now that he was laughing.